**Bruce King** earned h[...]
the early pioneers in [...]
attention of the gene[...]
the first people to open a multi-disciplinary natural
therapy clinic in London in the early sixties and was the
advisor on the Radio London Alternative Medicine
Advice Line, which was one of the most popular radio
advice lines at the time. He has also written regularly for
many national magazines on the subjects of slimming
and alternative medicine.

His work over more recent years led him to research
the power of the mind in helping people achieve results
that they thought were not possible in many different
fields of activity. His application of these same principles
to weight loss and weight control has resulted in what
can only be described as the most revolutionary and
successful approach ever to slimming.

*Also by Bruce King:*

**PSYCHO-SELLING**

# Psycho-Slimming

### Bruce King

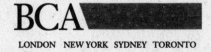

BCA

LONDON  NEW YORK  SYDNEY  TORONTO

This edition published 1995
by BCA
by arrangement with
HEADLINE BOOK PUBLISHING

CN 5352

Typeset by
Letterpart Limited, Reigate, Surrey

Printed and bound in Great Britain by
Cox & Wyman Ltd, Reading, Berks

Dedicated to my lovely wife Stephanie
– for all your help, patience and support.
Thank you!

# Contents

What should you eat? Your body knows best!
The primitive problem
Why does fat accumulate in certain places?
Rub your tummy away in ten minutes a day
The metabolism test
Psycho-Dynamic Programming exercises

## CHAPTER 3 – WEEK 3

Being positive is a key factor
The metabolic test results
How can you become more positive?
Defining your goals
Define your strategy to achieve this goal
Subconscious mind triggers
Exercise and your aim to achieve your perfect
    weight and shape
Psycho-Dynamic Programming exercises

## CHAPTER 4 – WEEK 4

It's your responsibility
Natural uppers and downers – the nutrient connection
The main food groups
Carbohydrate intolerance
Vitamins and minerals
Psycho-Slimming tips
Your progress to date
Your closest relationship – managing change
Psycho-Relative therapy
Psycho-Dynamic Programming exercises

# Foreword

**Psycho:** indicating the mind; psychological or mental processes.

**Slimming:** to reduce in size.

*Source – Collins*

**Psycho-Slimming:** Using your mind to achieve your perfect weight and shape – without dieting.

*Source – Bruce King*

Be honest with yourself. You are overweight and all the diets and exercise regimes you have tried in the past have failed. Let's face it, you would not have picked up this book in the first place if you had found the answer yet.

Well, now you have!

A quick glance through the following pages will reveal that there is not a great deal of dietary advice for you to follow. Dieting, in its recognised context, is not the answer. I know. For several years I ran one of the most successful slimming clinics in the UK and as well as putting our clients on very strict diets and exercise programmes in order to lose weight, we applied every other known technique to improve our results. To be honest with you, they did not work. Or rather, they did not work as well as I would have liked them to. Therefore, being the perfectionist that I am, I set out to find a method whereby everyone could lose weight and, more importantly, keep it off without effort.

I stopped giving people diets to follow a long time ago. In fact you, the reader, could probably teach me much more about the recent fad diets than I could ever teach you. I do however have something far more important to share with you.

I'm sure you know several people who eat as much as they want or overeat and never put on weight. The usual reason that is given is 'it's my metabolism'. You have also heard the expression 'it's all in the mind' applied to a variety of different situations and you have probably suspected that there is more than an element of truth to this. Well, you were right. It's not only their metabolism. It's their minds that keep them slim.

Frankly, it would be foolish of you not to put the principles I am going to teach you to the test. If you do, then at the end of this six-week course, you will be well on your way to your ideal weight – and keeping it there for life. What's more, you will have a lot more fun doing so and the lessons that you learn will also have a dramatic impact on many other aspects of your life and make it a lot more enjoyable in the future.

# Preface

As a former student of psychology, I was always fascinated by the mental processes which enabled some people to achieve aims and ambitions that other people might only dream about.

I therefore embarked on a long period of study to try to determine these hidden secrets and harness this power in order to provide everyone with the opportunity to achieve anything and everything that they wanted out of life.

It has taken me years to develop and perfect these techniques and involved me in hundreds of hours of study and many more practising and perfecting them. However, it is not going to take you that long to learn them and use them. The years of practice and my eagerness to pass this knowledge on to other people have enabled me to simplify these ideas so they can be taught in the shortest possible time and with the maximum effectiveness.

I call these techniques Psycho-Dynamic Programming, and by applying them over the next six weeks, you will quickly come to realise the power of your own mind and how you can use this power to achieve your perfect weight and shape and maintain it for ever.

How can I be so certain? Quite simply, I have taught these same techniques to hundreds of men and women in the past, and almost without exception, those who have followed my instructions have achieved precisely what it was that they wanted.

Let us take a few examples of what other people have achieved using Psycho-Dynamic Programming to illustrate the power of the human mind.

Susan X was a twenty-eight-year-old patient who came to visit me at my clinic. Susan was in a very bad way indeed. She had been drinking heavily for some years and was suffering from cirrhosis of the liver. She was extremely malnourished and, in the words of the last doctor she had seen, was only months away from an unpleasant death. I spent only one hour with Susan and explained her choices to her and what could be achieved if she was prepared to cooperate. Due to her fragile state, I was not sure that she would have even the little willpower necessary to put her Psycho-Dynamic Programming exercises into practice. However, she seemed keen to try and I gave her a very simple programme to start her off and asked her to come back and see me one week later or call me if she was having any difficulties.

Susan did not return the following week and I suspected the worst. About two years later I was walking down Regent Street and someone behind me called my name. I turned around, and standing behind me was one of the most attractive women I had seen in a long time. Yes, you guessed it. It was Susan. The change was, to say the least, remarkable.

We went off together and, in a quiet coffee house, Susan updated me on what had happened in her life since we last met. She told me that the short time I had spent with her and what I had taught her had done more for her than all the doctors and specialists she had seen in the past. She was completely cured, an absolute picture of health, and was now running her own very successful business. She apologised for not letting me know how she had been getting on but she had been so swept up with her new-found enthusiasm for life that she had literally dumped her past, including me, and moved on to better things. Needless to say, I was very happy for her.

Richard is another typical example. When I first met him, Richard had become one of life's losers. Physically he was a mess. He was fat, unfit, unhealthy and very unattractive. Mentally, he could cope with very little. He had held several jobs over the previous five years, each one more menial and poorly paid than the last. For the previous eighteen months he had been unemployed and had got to the point where he did not care if he ever worked again.

Six months later Richard was transformed. He looked terrific and felt better than he had felt for many years, both physically and mentally. He was the perfect weight for his height and was almost glowing with health. He was in regular employment and was taking a course at night school with a view to studying full time to become a lawyer. All due to the power of Psycho-Dynamic Programming.

And then there was Gladys. Twenty-three stone on a five foot two inches tall frame and so swaddled in fat that she had to be helped out of her car and into our clinic the first time that she attended, and in fact on several subsequent visits.

Gladys had circled the world in her quest for an answer to her weight problems and her food addictions. Fortunately she had the money to pay for these extravagant trips, and the money to waste, for none of these so-called 'miracle cures' had done her the least amount of good.

Gladys was cured of her food addictions and cravings within two weeks and gradually, over an eighteen-month period, got her weight down to a trim eleven stone by following the programme that we taught her. She looked like a 'million dollars' and felt the same.

Some years ago I was involved in teaching people to walk barefoot across beds of burning hot coals. The reason for these 'Fire-Walking Seminars' as they were called was to demonstrate that it was possible to achieve the seemingly impossible in a very short period of time. The Psycho-Dynamic Programming exercises consisted of a short period of deep relaxation, just like the exercise you will practise later, followed by a ten-minute period of visualising walking across the beds of glowing coals. Over fifty people were taught these simple visualisation techniques at each one of our seminars and very few did not have the confidence to walk across the fire at the end of the training. With few exceptions, there was not a blister in sight.

If the above examples seem almost miraculous, let me assure you that they are not. They are typical, everyday examples of what can be achieved using Psycho-Dynamic

Programming. Therefore they should encourage you to realise that, if such dramatic results can be achieved with such serious problems, your plans to achieve your perfect weight should be nothing more than a formality. And you will not have to walk on fire to achieve them!

# How to Use This Book

## WHAT IS WRONG WITH THE NORMAL 'DIET AND EXERCISE' APPROACH TO SLIMMING?

Almost every book that has ever been written before on the subject of slimming tends to concentrate entirely on dieting and exercise. I have nothing against that approach, except that, for most people, they don't achieve significant results and weight loss is rarely maintained.

It is all very well telling people what they should do, but it is another thing entirely to assist them to keep to a programme without any conscious effort on their part.

I recently came across some interesting statistics which indicated that of every one hundred people who go on the average weight loss programme, only eight of them achieve short-term success in meeting their ideal weight and less than one in a hundred has long-term success, meaning that for a year after they have been on a diet, they have maintained their ideal body weight. That is not very encouraging news for a public that spends literally hundreds of millions of pounds every year buying the products and services proffered by the 'Diet Industry'.

Let us take a closer look at those two words 'diet' and 'exercise'.

Even if you have never 'dieted' before, and I expect that most of you have, what images, thoughts and feelings does the word 'diet' conjure up? On the positive side there is the mental picture of you looking slimmer, fitter and more attractive to yourself and other people. However, the negative side of the picture is not so good. The word 'diet' is associated with deprivation, denying yourself foods that you would like to eat and replacing them with foods that you may not enjoy. 'Dieting' means eating less and the hunger pangs that often accompany this, as well as the tedious business of calorie counting.

What happens when you tell your friends that you are on a 'diet' again, probably for the third, fourth, fifth or however many times you have tried before? You must have seen their faces and read their expressions. The typical response, whether actually voiced out loud or not, is almost certainly a mixture of amusement, concern, pity, disbelief and possibly a touch of admiration. And flashing in neon lights is their subconscious reaction 'Oh no, not again. She'll never keep to it'. And these people are your friends!

Is it any wonder that, with all these negatives to cope with, the concept of dieting is almost doomed to failure before you even start?

What about 'exercise'? Once again, the positive picture is terrific. There you are, leaner, fitter, healthier, slimmer and bursting with energy and vitality. But what about the effort involved in getting yourself up that little bit earlier in the morning to do these exercises or finding the time and coping with the inconvenience of getting yourself down to the gym every day? How are you going to deal with taking the extra clothes to the exercise class with you so that you can change and get to the office on time? And how can you fit swimming into your busy schedule when the local pool doesn't open until three-thirty in the afternoon and you have to be at school to pick the children up at four?

It is hardly any wonder that nine out of ten people who make a conscious effort to put themselves on a strict exercise programme never even get started and of the one in ten who do, nine out of ten of those never keep to their original proposed schedule.

Well, from now on, any exercise programme that you do choose to pursue and I mean choose, not force it upon yourself, is going to be a pleasure for you and one which you will maintain for life. And as for 'dieting', you are never going to 'diet' again, you are never going to tell your friends you are going on a 'diet' again, and the word 'diet' will not be mentioned in this book again.

From now on you are on a different menu. It's called Psycho-Dynamic Programming. Your friends are going to notice a lot of things that are very different about you over the next few weeks and you are going to look better, feel better and lose weight without any of the negative feelings that you have associated with slimming in the past.

If, as a result of your Psycho-Dynamic Programming exercises, or PDP as we shall refer to it from now on, you feel inclined to eat less and use your body more in conjunction with these techniques, you should of course do so. Some adjustments to your eating habits and exercise programme, or lack of one, may well be necessary. The difference is that by the time your subconscious mind instructs you to make any changes,

3

the techniques you will have learned beforehand will increase the effectiveness of any regime that you select.

## BACKGROUND TO PSYCHO-DYNAMIC PROGRAMMING

I am going to ask you to do various things during your induction into the techniques of PDP that you may not be used to doing. The main reason for this is that you and I are both in a hurry. You are in a hurry to achieve your perfect weight in the simplest and most effective way, and I am eager to help you make it happen. I am therefore going to ask you to accept certain statements that I make almost without question.

I accept that under normal circumstances, it is every person's right to demand evidence before accepting anything, and I will give you some of this evidence as we go through the programme. However, how many times during any normal day do you take things at their face value without question? Let's be honest – we do what suits us most of the time. How often have you started on a crash slimming programme that you really knew did not make any sense whatsoever, but you decided to override your subconscious mind or 'gut feeling' and try it anyway?

Well, today is not a normal day. It is the first day of a six-week course that will change the way your body and your mind works for ever. And if the results I have achieved with people in the past are anything to go by, I suspect that by now, you are already beginning to realise that what I am saying makes an awful lot of sense and that it is in your interests to take what I am saying and what I am going to ask you to do at face value.

Your subconscious mind is already developing a feeling of trust and good faith in what I am sharing with you and we have barely started.

The detailed explanations for what I am going to ask you to do are available. However, to document them to your total satisfaction could occupy several shelves in the largest library. The techniques of PDP are distilled from research by some of the world's greatest psychologists, psychotherapists and experts from numerous other associated disciplines, and from studying and working with many of the most successful people from all walks of life. To ask you to read and digest this information to satisfy your curiosity and justify your involvement would defeat the object of the exercise.

I ask only that you give me approximately half an hour of your time, twice a day, every day, and practise the lessons that you will learn. The end will most definitely justify the means. No more of that dreaded word that I said we would not mention again. No more starvation or hunger pangs, no more constant, conscious attention to everything that you are eating and drinking and no more 'pain for gain'.

By the time you have finished this six-week course, you will be well on your way to achieving your perfect weight and shape and maintaining it for the rest of your life.

## ACHIEVING THE IMPOSSIBLE

Before we go any further, and because you are going to experience many things during the next six weeks that you previously thought were impossible, now is a good time to give you a simple demonstration of just how easy the impossible is to achieve.

Please carry out the following exercise now. It is the first of many that you will be doing during this programme.

**Exercise:**
*Stand up straight and hold your arms straight out in front of you and parallel to each other. Your fingers should be extended and pointing straight forward.*

*Now, keeping your legs and thighs rigid, twist your body from the waist and, keeping your arms in the same position in front of you, see how far you can swivel your upper body to the left. When it is impossible for you to twist any more, note what object your left fingers are pointing at and then return to your original position.*

*Now take a note of a point somewhat further round than your fingers were able to point towards when you did that first part of the exercise, some point that was impossible for you to reach before.*

*Now start again in the same position and swivel your upper body again until your fingers are pointing to that impossible position.*

*You did it, didn't you? You achieved the impossible!*

## THE SUBCONSCIOUS MIND
The human brain is an extremely complex organ but for the sake of simplicity, let's just divide it into the two parts that I have already mentioned, the conscious and the subconscious mind. This is probably not a new concept to anybody.

The conscious mind is the one that you are in control

of. It is the analytical part of the brain, the one that talks to you in words all of the time. It is the one you hear very clearly in your head whenever you are thinking and it is the part that you frequently argue with and which creates confusion, indecision and unhappiness.

The subconscious mind is the part that very few people ever listen to regularly, but is in truth the part which controls so many of your decision-making processes and the way you react to people and different situations. Everyone has experienced having a 'gut feeling'. That's the subconscious mind. It is rarely wrong because its knowledge is based on millions of experiences that you are unable to remember with your conscious mind. I am sure that you can recall many occasions when you made the wrong decision about something quite important and afterwards have said to yourself, 'I wish I had trusted my gut feelings'.

The first important point I want you to accept is that you cannot convince or teach your inner being, the 'real' you, by instructing the conscious mind. Real learning and total change can only take place when your mind is at least somewhere between the conscious and the subconscious mode. It is only when you take in information in this state that the subconscious mind will absorb the new knowledge and allow you to use this knowledge instead of resisting and rejecting it.

Of course some people can overcome the subconscious mind by using a tremendous amount of willpower. However, this programme that you are taking part in is designed to make everything you want to achieve happen for you as easily as possible without having to rely on willpower and its relatively poor success rate.

When was the last time you said to yourself or your conscious mind, 'I am going on a "xxxx" from tomorrow?' No matter how positive you were as you said it, I guarantee that a little voice deep down inside said 'no you are not', 'you will never keep to it', or 'it won't work'. That was the subconscious mind in action, telling you that, on the basis of everything that it has learned since the day that you were born, it does not agree with your conscious mind. And the subconscious mind almost always wins.

You must also accept that you cannot learn the techniques of PDP by reading a chapter quickly when going to work on the train, in a short coffee break, whilst grabbing a hurried meal, or in fact at any time when your mind is not fully capable of absorbing the information you need to know. Therefore, for just a few weeks, accept the simple discipline that you must set aside some private time in order for you to benefit from this programme.

## YOU MUST READ ONLY ONE OF THE FOLLOWING CHAPTERS EACH WEEK

And practise what you have learned during the week in conjunction with the simple PDP exercises that I will teach you. Of course I don't expect you not to have a quick flick through the following pages and get an overview of what you have just invested in, but after that, if you seriously want to achieve your perfect weight and shape, you must follow my instructions to the letter.

You must also accept that the fastest way to make things happen is to make sure that your subconscious mind, as well as your conscious mind, knows clearly what it is you want to happen, and that the fastest way to get this message through to the subconscious mind is to visualise exactly what it is that you want. Once you have put a clear mental picture into the subconscious mind, you need not worry any longer about how things will happen – you must just accept that they most definitely will. This is the fundamental rule on which all PDP techniques are based.

## MONITORING YOUR PROGRESS

At the end of each chapter of this programme you will find a chart which you will complete at the end of each week. This is designed to aid you in monitoring the improvements that will inevitably take place over the course of each week and subsequent weeks. They are easy to complete and will take you literally no more than a few minutes. They are there for your benefit, and will be a striking illustration of the changes that are taking place within you, not only relating to your actual weight, but also numerous other 'feel good factors' that will make you look better and feel better than you have ever looked or felt before.

If these results do not satisfy you and make you feel increasingly good about yourself each week, there can be only one reason for this. You will not have been following my instructions.

I expect you to read each chapter twice during the week, once at the beginning of the week and again halfway through it. You may also read it every day if you feel that this helps you; many people do. You must also carry out the exercise on page 14 and repeat this same exercise twice daily, together with those others that are taught to you in each of the following chapters.

## PSYCHO-DYNAMIC PROGRAMMING EXERCISES

Before you carry out the first of your PDP exercises, I want to explain to you the importance of the breathing pattern you are going to use in the first five minutes of this exercise. This breathing pattern is going to be different from the normal breathing pattern that you use for the remaining fifteen minutes.

You may often have heard the expression 'the breath of life' and there is a great deal more to this than you think, particularly with regard to your aim to achieve your perfect weight and shape.

If you were to stop breathing, you would die. This is quite obvious. If you only half breathe, you are only half alive. That statement needs a little more explanation.

Proper breathing has as much of a positive effect on your physical and mental well-being as any other form of therapy. On the physical side, breathing enlivens the body. It introduces vital oxygen into the bloodstream which is then carried round to all the millions of cells throughout your body. This oxygen improves the health of the cells and enhances the electrical activity in those cells. Oxygen makes them act and react more quickly when your body needs them to. It means that your body acts more efficiently to keep you healthy and will also help produce the results that your subconscious mind wants it to produce, such as losing weight.

Breathing also helps the body to circulate lymph fluid around your system. Lymph is a living fluid that surrounds all the cells in your body and in fact you have more lymph circulating in your system than you have blood. The main function of the lymph fluid is to remove all the toxins and poisonous wastes that build up in your body as a result of what you eat and how the body breaks it down into essential nutrients and waste products. If your lymphatic system is not working properly, you are being slowly poisoned and nothing ever works quite as it should.

You understand the importance of the heart; the moment this stops beating and pumping blood around, you die. The lymphatic system has no such pump to move lymph fluid around and it is dependent on other methods to maintain its circulation around your body. The first is breathing and the second is movement.

Most people have so much conscious and subconscious tension in their lives that they find it almost physically impossible to breathe properly without making a conscious effort. Even then, many find it difficult at first. Their breathing is shallow and ineffective.

Five minutes of good breathing exercises, twice a day, does wonders for the lymphatic system, helps to relax and release tension and educates the lungs to start breathing properly again. It helps to get all those accumulated poisons out of your system and, apart from assisting you in achieving your perfect weight and shape, it will make you feel a lot better in many other ways.

After the five minutes of breathing exercises, I will then guide you through a fifteen-minute pre-programming and relaxation exercise. Just follow my instructions and allow yourself to let go. You will then drift into a state where your subconscious mind will be able to absorb new ideas rapidly and without any effort on your part.

Try this first exercise now and then re-read these first few pages. You will immediately notice how much more easily you absorb the information, and tomorrow it will be as fresh in your mind as if you had just read it.

Just one more word before you start: let's not confuse this with brainwashing. Brainwashing is something that is forced upon you. You volunteered to achieve your perfect weight and shape and that is precisely what you are going to do. Having said that, I can think of a lot of good reasons for people having their brains washed once in a while and getting rid of some of those cobwebs that have been holding them back from achieving the success that they deserve.

*Exercise:*
First of all, make absolutely certain that you are not going to be disturbed for the next half-hour. Take the telephone off the hook or switch on your answering machine if you have one. If there is anybody in the house or office or wherever you intend to carry out these exercises, make sure they understand your absolute need for privacy and that they will cooperate with you.

Now sit in a comfortable chair, make sure that you can see your watch or a clock easily, read the rest of these instructions and then just put them into practice.

For the first minutes of this exercise, I want you to close your eyes and concentrate on breathing in the following manner.

Breathe from your stomach and feel the breath coming up into your chest. Breathe in for two seconds, hold the breath for six seconds and breathe out again for four seconds. As your lungs get stronger and more elastic over the next few weeks, extend the amount of time that you breathe in, hold and breathe out, but always keep them in the same ratios. Do this part of the breathing exercise for five minutes.

When this five minutes is up, I want you to continue breathing as you would normally do and concentrate on relaxing and letting the tension go from every part of your body.

You start with your toes and go up the legs part by part

*until you have reached and relaxed your buttocks. Feel the tension draining from each part of your body before you go on to the next. Then do the same with your arms, starting with your fingers and working up until you end with your shoulders fully relaxed. All this time I would like you to breathe steadily and gently. When your shoulders are fully relaxed, start at the top of your head, your scalp, work down the back of your neck and your back down to your waist. Next, make sure your forehead is relaxed, then all the muscles of your face, particularly your jaw.*

*Finally, allow your chest muscles to relax. After a little practice and probably no more than a few days, this whole process will take no more than five minutes. Then, for the next ten minutes, I want you to do absolutely nothing but concentrate on the sound of your breathing. Please realise that it is inevitable that from time to time you will stop concentrating on your breathing and will find that your mind is drifting off in different directions. That is fine. All you need do when you realise this is happening is to go back to concentrating on your breathing. Remember that you do this for a full fifteen minutes and if you need to check your watch or the clock, only open one eye. This keeps the subconscious mind focused.*

*This first part of your mental exercises is the pre-programming or subconscious entry stage.*

*At the end of this part of the exercise, keeping your eyes closed, I want you to sit there for another ten minutes and do nothing but visualise your body exactly as you would like it to be in the future.*

*This is very serious and you should not compromise. No matter how unrealistic your ideal figure may seem to you right now, it is possible to achieve it and that is precisely how you must visualise yourself. See yourself as you are going to be in the future if this programme is going to work for you as well as I say it will. Picture yourself exactly as it will look to you when you have arrived at your perfect weight and shape.*

*Read these instructions one more time so that you fully understand them, put them into practice and I will catch up with you later in Chapter One.*

## SUMMARY OF KEY POINTS

- Read only one chapter a week and read each chapter at least twice during the week. Read it every day if you wish. If you do not have the time every day then just read the summary of key points.
- Practise your PDP exercises every day, twice a day, and precisely as you have been instructed.
- Real learning only takes place when the mind is somewhere between the conscious and subconscious mode.
- The fastest way to make things happen is to put a clear picture into your subconscious mind of what it is that you want to happen. The subconscious mind will then make it happen for you. This process is known as Psycho-Dynamic Programming, referred to from now on as PDP.
- Please remember that all that I am asking from you is half an hour, twice a day, every day for the next six weeks. During these half-hour sessions, all that I shall be asking you to do is a simple series of mental exercises. I am asking very little of you compared to what any other slimming programme has demanded of you before and am promising you dramatically better results.
- I care passionately that you keep to this programme and achieve the results that you want. Give us both a chance!

# CHAPTER ONE

# Your Beautiful Mind –
# Your Beautiful Body

The first thing that I would like to do is to congratulate you!

You obviously read a few pages of this book before deciding to purchase it, heard about it from a friend or heard me being interviewed about it on the radio or television. .Whichever it was, you must have realised or been told that this book was going to make a major change to your life.

So congratulations – most people find it so difficult to make a dramatic change to any aspect of their lives. In fact most people actually make very few major changes in their lives at all. They generally just tend to go on as they have always done before and, mostly, people react when they are forced to and rarely change very much out of choice. Most of the time you are controlled by your environment and are at the mercy of everything that is going on around you. Some psychiatrists call this the 'victim syndrome'.

Whenever you do try to make a conscious decision to change something, you almost certainly try to do so with

18

your conscious mind. A voice in your head keeps up a constant dialogue and tries to rationalise your decision for you and allow the change to take place. Unfortunately it is up against some very stiff competition and yes – you probably guessed it – the competition is the subconscious mind.

The subconscious mind has stored hundreds of thousands of items of information within it over the years, all of them based on your past experiences. The subconscious mind always thinks it knows best. It is not always right but it has been programmed by you to think and act the way that it does.

The other problem with trying to outsmart your subconscious mind is that you and it are probably not speaking in the same language. Whenever you try to make a positive decision to change something, you almost certainly speak to your conscious mind in words. That is the basis of most forms of communication and so it seems logical to talk silently to ourselves when trying to rationalise and decide on any course of action. But is it logical? The answer is no! Verbal communication is only a very small part of the story, so let us take a closer look at how we communicate with ourselves and other people.

## HOW DO WE COMMUNICATE?

The basic method of communication between most people is verbal language and that is probably the major reason why communication between people breaks down so often. You may speak with words but you do not necessarily receive the messages with them. Different people will receive different messages communicated by the same words depending on how their subconscious minds interpret them when they are received.

Words may be the primary communicator but these are translated by your mind into one of three different modalities.

The first is Auditory, in which case you hear the words and all the other sounds associated with the subject that you are discussing. You hear the message clearly and often are listening to your own internal conversation at the same time.

The second mode is the Visual mode. When you are operating in a visual mode your mind will paint a picture with the words and it is the picture that will give meaning to the communication.

The third mode is known as the Kinaesthetic mode. This involves all the other senses that make you feel something as opposed to hear it or see it. This could include a sense of touch or smell but mainly consists of a number of strong feelings inside you to which you can relate.

Unless you can communicate with another person in the mode in which they are most likely to receive the message, your message may become very confused to them and may not be understood at all.

Let me illustrate this with some simple examples. Let us suppose that you are trying to communicate to a friend how you felt about a beautiful display of flowers that you had just seen. You describe how the flower display looked. You may be talking to them in terms of colour, shape and size. However, this person does not think of flowers in terms of a picture. To them, flowers have some form of deep emotional attachment and they can only understand them and appreciate them in terms of smell and the emotions that they associate with them. You will not be conveying the same picture or message.

Or suppose that you are proposing a day out with a friend and you run through a list of things that you would like to do and places that you would like to visit. Having outlined your plans to your friend, you are now about to ask them for their opinion.

If your friend's dominant receptive mode is visual and you ask them, 'How do you feel about that?', they will find it hard to reply or communicate their response. You will have confused their thinking process by communicating in a kinaesthetic way.

On the other hand, if you had asked, 'How does that fit into your picture of our day together?' or, 'How do you see that working out?' you would get an immediate and clear response.

If your friend's primary receptive mode was auditory and you asked them, 'How do you see that as a day out?' they would once again get a confused message and find it difficult to answer. Do you get the picture? Do you understand what I am saying? Does that feel right to you?

Your subconscious mind stores information and acts on information in all three of these different ways. Therefore in order to communicate with it properly, it is essential that the communication takes place on all these different levels. The simplest and most effective way of doing this is through the techniques of Psycho-Dynamic Programming.

## HOW DO PSYCHO-DYNAMIC PROGRAMMING EXERCISES WORK?

You now know that the PDP exercises that you are going to carry out every day are split into two parts. The first part is the pre-programming stage and takes twenty minutes. Without this pre-programming exercise, it is not possible for you to access the subconscious mind and the new messages that we want to put in there would not be readily accepted.

Having said that, by the end of six weeks, you will no longer need to go through this twenty-minute exercise in order to access your subconscious mind. By that time, you will have set up an entry route and I will show you a much faster way to access this at the end of this programme. Do not think you can do it now. It is only by regular practice of these techniques for six weeks that this shortened technique will work for you in the future.

Let me give you some brief background information into the way that the pre-programming exercises work.

You have all heard of meditation and know that this has been practised for thousands of years by many people from all races and religions. Many exceptional mental talents and abilities have been credited to the techniques of meditation.

Meditation is simply a form of deep, controlled relaxation, as are the pre-programming exercises that you will do. Scientific experiments have proven that the deep relaxation techniques are the key to various other mental strategies such as accelerated learning, visualisation, mental problem solving, self-healing and of course the state of self-hypnosis which in itself creates a state of hyper-receptivity and hyper-suggestibility.

One particular scientific experiment that took place compared the learning and thinking abilities of a group of people who were taught a series of lessons in normal classroom conditions compared to another group of equal IQ who were taught the same lessons in a darkened room, with no distractions, and after a period of pre-programming such as you will do.

The results were dramatically different. Most important of all was the fact that the more difficult subsequent tests became, the better the results were of the pre-programmed group.

Once you have been through the pre-programming stage, it then becomes a simple matter to put new messages into your subconscious mind, and providing that you communicate these messages in all three sensory modalities, the subconscious mind will be able to absorb your instructions.

The last thing that you need to know is that with one further simple exercise which will take no more than five seconds, it then becomes possible to lock that message in so that it then has a strong and overriding effect on any of the bad messages that have been stored in the past. You will be taught this technique soon and at the appropriate time.

Enough of the long words and scientific explanations – the fact is that we have a simple, effective and virtually guaranteed method of helping you to achieve your perfect weight and shape.

Most of you have no idea of how a nuclear electric power station produces electricity but you have no qualms about turning on the lights, the television or the radio. I doubt that you understand the workings of the internal combustion engine but you get into your car and drive it away without thinking about it. I certainly have no idea of how my word processor works, but I have no problems in accepting that it will do the job that I ask of it.

Therefore, please take my word and trust that Psycho-Dynamic Programming and the other techniques that you will learn will definitely work for you. Let us now proceed.

## YOUR BEAUTIFUL MIND – YOUR BEAUTIFUL BODY

The inside workings of your body are incredible: all those millions of cells within your mind controlling all those billions of cells making up the different organs, muscles, and tissues throughout your body; all the complex chemical reactions that are taking place all day and every day. What an extraordinary, wondrous and beautiful system. Well, most of that seems to take fairly good care of itself, given the right nutrition and a moderate amount of exercise. What you are really concerned about, and the reason that you bought this book, is the packaging – what it all looks like from the outside. So let's take a look at your packaging.

## YOU ARE ALREADY BEAUTIFUL

There is already a great deal about you, inside and outside, that is very beautiful. Yes – you, all of you. There is not one single person who does not have an awful lot of wonderful features about them. They could be physical attributes such as your hair, your lips, your ears, your neck. It could be your toes, your ankles, your hands, arms, breasts or any number of things. They may not all fit together quite as you would like them to just yet, but nevertheless they are there.

What about your personality? That changes frequently, doesn't it? Sometimes you are feeling really good about something and it affects everything and everyone around you. Sometimes you are feeling down and this shows too. There are many different aspects to your personality. Are you fun, caring, do you relate well to other people and do they come to you for counselling or advice? Do they value your opinions? These are also beautiful features and they are reflected in the way you look and the way you carry yourself.

There are a lot more beautiful things about you, and you know it. Do not let the fact that you feel you are overweight and out of shape detract from these.

### Exercise:

*Before you go any further, I want you to get a blank sheet of paper and I would like you to make a list. I want you to put down in writing every single thing about you that you feel good about. You may like to do this with a close friend, partner, spouse or other appropriate person that you have trust and faith in. It may even be someone else who has bought this book and is starting out on the same journey as you. We often find that people have more fun on our programme if they work through it in groups, and they often get better and faster results. You may choose to do this also.*

*So whether you are doing it alone, or with that appropriate person or group of people, start with your physical attributes and take each part of your body in isolation. You should have a mirror close at hand so that you can see the parts that are not visually accessible without one, or use your friend for these areas.*

*Start with your toes and piece by piece, work your way up your body. Be totally honest with yourself, be flattering and do not be embarrassed. There is nothing to be embarrassed about. If you think your toes are beautiful – write it down descriptively – 'I have beautiful toes'. If your feet are slim and pretty but your ankles are larger than you would wish, ignore your ankles. Write down – 'I have beautiful slim feet'. Do this from the tip of your toes to the top of your scalp and do not leave out one single thing. If it is your breasts, your shoulders, your elbows, your lips, nose, ears or anything else, write it down. Please remember, though, I want only positive things written down, all the parts of you that maybe you had not thought about before, but on close examination, are actually very nice when taken in isolation.*

*When you have done this, I want you to look at the many aspects of your personality that make up this beautiful person that is you.*

*First of all your relationships. Not only your close ones, but relationships with all the people in your life. There are a lot of attractive features about your personality and how you behave with and towards other people that are really exceptional and these need to go on the list too.*

*What about your career, whether it is as a home-keeper or if you have an outside career? What do you contribute to this that is something to be proud of and which makes you feel good when you think about it? Write that down too, please. Anything that you can think of that enhances your self-image should go down on what is likely to become a very long list.*

*When you have finished this list, read it through a couple of times to remind yourself again. Do not cross anything out. If you write it down the first time it was right to be there. I know how difficult it may be for you to accept any form of praise, let alone self-praise. I know how much easier it is to criticise yourself, but you deserve self-praise and recognition much more than you deserve criticism, so let go and enjoy it.*

## WHAT IS YOUR PERFECT WEIGHT AND SHAPE?

So what about the packaging? What about your weight, your shape and your size? How beautiful are you and how much more beautiful can you be and do you want to be?

By the end of this, your first week of working with me, I want you to be in a position where you have finally decided, once and for ever, just what you want your perfect weight and shape to be. And I mean you, not some other person's vision.

If you are in a relationship with someone who claims to love you but would prefer you to try and become the impossible dream of their perfect man or woman, and you know it is impossible, then maybe you should be changing the relationship. It is not possible to shrink bone, muscle and tissue and not fair on you for someone to expect you to try.

At the end of this first week I want you to know precisely how you want to look, how much you want to weigh and how you want to feel. I want you to be able to experience this with all of the senses that we discussed earlier and I want you to be so clear about it in your mind that if I were to wake you at two in the morning from a deep sleep, you could give me a perfect description of how you are going to be in the not too distant future.

Now, just how is that going to be in terms of your weight and shape? I suspect that by the end of this week it is not going to be quite as you imagine it right now.

*Exercise:*

*Before you make any firm decisions on how much you want to weigh and how you want to look in the future, I want you to take a careful look at the overall picture you present now. That does not mean that I want you to picture yourself as you are first thing in the morning with no make-up and your hair all over the place, slouched in front of a mirror. Some of the most voluptuous, beautiful film stars I have met look absolutely dreadful first thing in the morning. And as for the ultra-slim models that parade the catwalks of the fashion world draped in those expensive designer clothes, I can assure you that in most cases, the reality first thing in the morning leaves an awful lot to be desired.*

*No, I want you to picture yourself as you are at your very best, dressed for a night out, or for a day out with a friend on a more casual occasion, but after you have taken more than just a little trouble with yourself. That is, after all, how you can choose to be at any time.*

*If you happen to live in a particularly sunny part of the country and spend a lot of time around a pool, scantily clad in a swimsuit, in spite of the recent skin cancer scares, and that is where you need to be to feel the most comfortable with your weight and size, then picture yourself at your very best in that situation.*

*The terrible thing about assessing your own looks and beauty is that you tend to examine yourself as if you were under a huge magnifying glass, but yours is a most unusual one. It magnifies the bad points and for some strange reason, it diminishes the good ones. So how do you think you really look when you stop the extreme self-criticism and look at yourself through someone else's eyes?*

I am not asking you to make any decision yet. This will come quite naturally by the end of the week and as a result of your PDP exercises. But I do want you to give some more realistic thought to your perfect weight and size now.

Just how much weight do you really need and want to lose in order to achieve your perfect weight and shape?

## PLEASE BE REALISTIC

Whilst I am able to help you achieve your perfect weight, neither I nor you can perform miracles, so please keep this in mind when deciding how it is that you want to be in the future. If you have a very large bone structure and you expect or want to look ultra-thin, I am afraid this is just not possible and you already know that. If that is the case, then trying to remove more than just excess fat in an attempt to achieve the impossible is almost certain to make you less attractive than you may be now. It is just as likely that you may decide that you need to take off more weight in some places and put some on in others in order to achieve that slightly larger, bustier and curvier figure that was so admired by men in the not too distant past and is still admired by a good many men and women today.

And what if the opposite is the case and you have a very tiny frame on which to support your outer covering?

Once again, there is only so much you should want to achieve and only so much that is possible to achieve without spoiling what is already probably very attractive to someone you know.

So be realistic, be sensible and accept that if you have a lot of weight to lose, you are obviously going to have to eat less. If you want to develop more curves in the right places and get a better, trimmer, firmer shape, accept that some exercise is going to be necessary and that your subconscious mind is going to take care of all this for you. When, by the end of this week, you have decided precisely what it is that you want to look like in the future, I shall help put you and your subconscious mind on autopilot so that you reach your destination as quickly and simply as possible.

This is your first week on the programme and that really is all I want you to do for this week apart from your PDP exercises. If this does not seem like a lot of progress now, it certainly will by the end of this week. The way you will feel about having defined your future perfect weight and shape at the end of this week is something that cannot be described by me. Only you can experience it.

### Elizabeth's experience

Elizabeth was a patient of mine. She described her experience as one of such enormous relief that that alone was worth a million dollars. She had been constantly battling to lose an extra ten pounds for years in order to look good in a swimsuit that she wore for only two weeks a year. The really exciting thing for her was that once she had decided that she did not want to lose those few pounds any more, she looked brighter and more beautiful than she had ever done before.

If by the end of this week and as a result of these PDP exercises you have defined your perfect weight and you decide that you are perfectly happy the way you are, then you will not need to continue with this programme. If that is the case, then put this book away or give it to a friend and go ahead and enjoy your life as you are now. You will be feeling as good about yourself as Elizabeth did, and rightly so.

If you are already on some sort of exercise programme and you are happy with it, then please keep it up. The same goes for any sensible eating plan. I will deal with these aspects of your programme in later Chapters. For the next week I just want you to carry out your PDP exercises and get this clear picture of the future 'You' deep down into your subconscious mind.

One last thing before I instruct you on this week's PDP exercises. Do not tell anyone other than your closest friend or appropriate person that you are undertaking this six-week programme. It is an unfortunate fact of life that most people like to see other people fail. It makes them feel better about their own failures. Do not set yourself up as a target for other people to knock down. You will have all the support and power that is necessary to achieve your perfect weight and shape from me and the incredible resources within you that we are going to unearth together. Keep this programme to yourself and let others wonder why you are looking and feeling so good.

## YOUR PSYCHO-DYNAMIC PROGRAMMING EXERCISES FOR THIS WEEK

*These exercises need to be carried out as early as is possible for you in the morning, bearing in mind your own commitments and timetable, and again at some time in the evening, preferably before you go to bed but not in bed. If this is not a convenient time, then do the second set of exercises when you get home in the early evening; or if you look after a home and children and the only time you get to yourself is before school is out, then late afternoon is also fine. As long as the routine for these PDP exercises is established and can be maintained, you can suit yourself.*

### Morning PDP Exercises
*First of all, carry out your twenty-minute breathing, relaxation and pre-programming exercise. When you have completed this, keep your eyes closed and spend the next ten minutes repeating the following statement over and over again to yourself, without speaking the words out loud.*

*'I (your name) am in the process of achieving and maintaining my perfect weight and this will be mine to keep for ever. My success is guaranteed.'*

### Evening PDP Exercises
*Once again, go through the pre-programming exercise.*

*When you have completed this, I want you to picture yourself clearly in precisely the way that you wish to be in the future. Whatever you have decided is your perfect weight and shape for the future, experience it in your mind as if it has already happened and feel it with all your senses. See yourself as you will be. Feel how it feels with as much intensity as you possibly can. Hear your inner voice complimenting you and the voices of others with whom you are sharing this experience and programme.*

*At any time during this ten-minute visualisation exercise and whenever you feel really good about how you are experiencing the feelings, touch the tip of your little finger against the tip of your thumb and exert a little pressure. This technique will lock the picture into your subconscious mind from where it will be accessed whenever you need it, and without you having to do it consciously.*

These exercises are very simple and you should have no difficulty in achieving the mental pictures that are required. They will also get easier every day.

You may also change your mind during the course of this week as to how you would like to be in the future. This is fine and is all part of the process. By the end of this first week your perfect weight and size will be truly established in your subconscious and conscious mind.

## EATING DISORDERS
If you are one of the many people who are troubled by one of the various eating disorders, please turn to the section in the appendix which deals with special situations. There are additional exercises there which could

help you to overcome your condition. Please incorporate these extra exercises into your daily routine.

If they fail to help, please do seek suitable medical advice on a one-to-one basis but please also continue with the rest of this programme. It will be a valuable adjunct to any other therapy that you may need to undertake.

## SUMMARY OF KEY POINTS

- Your subconscious mind currently controls almost everything that you do and is your major obstacle to change. Psycho-Dynamic Programming can enable you to communicate with your subconscious mind and to take control.

- You must communicate with the subconscious mind with visual, auditory and kinaesthetic communication techniques.

- Your body is already beautiful in many ways. Make a list of all your best attributes, physical, mental and others. Do this with a friend or other appropriate person if you wish.

- Day by day, during your PDP exercise programmes, develop a clear picture of how you want to look in the future. Be realistic, sensible, but as ambitious as you wish. If, by the end of this week, you have decided that you are already your perfect weight and shape, put this book away or give it to a friend and enjoy yourself as you are.

- Carry out your morning and evening PDP exercises.

- If your subconscious mind is encouraging you to eat less and more sensibly this week, it is fine for you to follow these inner instructions.

- If you also feel inclined to start getting some more exercise, that is fine also. However, do not force yourself into any exercise programme that you could not or do not want to maintain. Just walking up the occasional flight of stairs instead of taking the lift will do fine.

- If you have any form of eating disorder, turn to the relevant pages in the appendix and carry out the additional PDP exercises. If these do not help, please seek medical advice but continue with this programme.
- Complete the progress monitor chart at the end of this week.

## PROGRESS MONITOR – PLEASE COMPLETE AT THE END OF THE LAST DAY OF THE WEEK

**Instructions:**

Place a tick in the relevant column alongside each of the following questions. Do not think about your answers for too long – your initial reaction to each question will be the most accurate answer.

**Compared to the start of this programme:**

| | worse | the same | better | much better | very much better | totally satisfied |
|---|---|---|---|---|---|---|
| How do you feel about your weight and shape now? | | | | | | |
| How do you think other people feel about your weight and shape now? | | | | | | |
| How do you feel about yourself as a person, taking into account factors such as your confidence, personality, sense of humour and ability to relate to and communicate with other people? | | | | | | |
| If you are in a close relationship with another person, how do you feel about this relationship now? | | | | | | |
| If you are in a close relationship with another person, how do you think that other person feels about this relationship now? | | | | | | |
| How do you feel about your confidence and ability to achieve your perfect weight and shape in the future and keep it there for ever? | | | | | | |
| How do you feel about being able to eat less, and more sensibly and nutritiously, in the future? | | | | | | |
| How do you feel about your ability to maintain any form of general exercise routine in the future? | | | | | | |

**My weight at the beginning of this programme was:**

# CHAPTER TWO

## WEEK TWO

# The Body–Mind Connection

**INNER THOUGHTS CREATE INNER ACTION**
Every single thought that your subconscious and your conscious mind have also creates an action or reaction within your physical body. There is no exception to this rule. The more powerful the subconscious message becomes, the more powerful the effect on your physical body. Once you have come to terms with this statement you will realise even more the power of Psycho-Dynamic Programming.

Let us take a simple, everyday example to illustrate this.

You mentally decide that you want to have a cup of black coffee. The instant that decision is taken, your body goes into action. Your stomach and other parts of your body begin to anticipate the reaction to this liquid intake. Your taste buds become active in anticipation, your stomach may rumble a little and you may automatically lick your lips.

A whole series of other physical actions are now necessary in order for you to prepare this beverage. You need to walk over to the cupboard, take out the coffee, fill the percolator with water, switch on the electricity, take out a cup and saucer or mug, and carry out a whole host of other physical tasks in order to reach the final conclusion when you sit down and enjoy your drink. Most of these actions you now carry out automatically, in fact almost subconsciously, because you have done them so many times before. However, not one of these actions can be undertaken without a whole series of chemical reactions and nerve reactions taking place in your body.

In order for you simply to lift a finger, a small group of cells in your brain must be activated and send messages to several other parts of the brain. These messages then have to go down various other pathways and activate nerves, muscles and tendons to perform these tasks for you. Every one of these messages is accompanied by chemical changes in the various parts of the body that need to be activated in order for that finger to be moved. The nerves which transmit these messages send tiny electrical impulses from one nerve cell to another, all the way from your brain down to your little finger in order for this one tiny movement to take place.

That is a very simplified explanation, but it does demonstrate how much has to go on in that beautiful body of yours in order for you to get a cup of coffee prepared. Several other millions of tiny impulses and chemical changes take place throughout your system as each action and reaction takes place and when you finally get around to drinking the coffee itself, the smell, taste and the reaction of the liquid and caffeine within your system provokes several million other actions and reactions, all of which have to be fed back to the brain in order that it can maintain control. It really is quite an incredible procedure.

For every conscious or subconscious thought or action that takes place, another series of actions and reactions take place. So how can we use these natural systems that are in place to help you achieve your perfect weight and shape?

*Exercise:*
*Let us take another very different example.*

*Sit down in an upright chair and think about something that makes you feel really unhappy. Concentrate on this and try and put yourself in that frame of mind. Allow your body to get into the posture that it would be in when you feel that way. Allow your face muscles to form the expression that you would have at the time and allow that sinking, miserable feeling to take you over. Are you feeling bad?*

*Now, sit up straight, pull your shoulders back, lift your chin up and give a big smile! Are you feeling better? I know you are. Now repeat this exercise again and note how easy it is to change the way that you feel, just by changing your posture and the expression on your face.*

What is happening here is quite straightforward and yet is a very powerful demonstration of the body–mind connection.

Your subconscious mind has been programmed over the years to associate your posture and your facial expressions with a particular state of mind that you are in at the time. If you slump your shoulders and look unhappy, your body will carry out millions of tiny chemical and nerve reactions and make sure that you feel how you look. The reverse is also true. When you are feeling really good about yourself, for whatever reason, your body makes you adopt the posture and facial expressions that it associates with that particular set of thoughts, and once again it does this by causing a whole different set of chemical and nerve reactions.

If you ever again find yourself bursting into tears because of something that has made you so unhappy, try pulling back your shoulders, lifting your chin up and forcing a grin. You will not be able to do both together. You will either find it impossible to lift your chin and smile or you will be able to do so, in which case you will find it almost impossible to continue crying. Try this with yourself or someone else when the situation arises. I have often been able to change my children from a state of total misery into laughing hyenas in the space of a few seconds with this body–mind reaction.

## ACT AS IF YOU ALREADY ARE

Acting as if you have already achieved your perfect weight and shape is one of the most powerful PDP techniques that you can use. When you start to act as you expect to be in the future, your subconscious mind sets in motion thousands and thousands of chemical and nerve reactions in your body to support your intentions, just as we described before.

So powerful is this technique that if this was the only exercise you ever carried out in this whole six-week programme, you would eventually achieve your perfect weight and shape. As part of our overall programme and with all the other things that you are doing, you cannot fail.

So how would you act now if you were already your perfect weight and shape? Well obviously, if you are a size

43

eighteen, I'm not expecting you to try and slip into a size fourteen dress just yet, but there are an awful lot of other things that you can do to trick your subconscious mind into getting your body to help you lose weight that much faster. So just precisely what would you do if you were already your perfect weight and shape?

Would you take more care of your appearance than you do now? Would you walk differently, talk differently, show more confidence in your approach to other people around you? Would your posture be any different? Would you hold your chin up higher, smile more and be more friendly and communicative with other people? Would you get more involved in other activities if you felt better about your appearance and felt that you were more attractive to those of your own and the opposite sex?

Obviously every person would react differently, and therefore it is up to you to decide how you will act and behave from now.

Does this all seem a little daunting and possibly too much to handle? I thought it might be, and so I am going to make it a lot easier for you.

*Exercise:*
The following PDP exercise is going to empower you to be
now as you will be when you are your perfect weight and
size. And we are going to select the most difficult set of
circumstances that you can possibly imagine. Once you can
easily overcome this situation, you will be able to act this
way under any circumstances from now on.

## PROGRAMMING YOUR SUBCONSCIOUS MIND TO ACT AS IF YOU ARE ALREADY YOUR PERFECT WEIGHT AND SHAPE

This Psycho-Dynamic Programming exercise is done in
three simple stages.

### Stage One

Clearly identify the situation in which you feel most
uncomfortable about your weight and shape. For example,
it may be a time when you have to take your clothes off in
front of some other person; it may be when you walk into
a room full of strangers or when you first walk down to the
swimming pool on holiday. Close your eyes and create a
picture of you doing whatever is so uncomfortable for you
to do.

You may feel more able to create this picture as if it were a
snapshot, or you may find it easier to create it as if it were
part of a film. In either case, create it as brightly and
vividly and in as much detail as you possibly can. If it will
have more impact on you as a black and white picture or
film, create it in black and white. If the picture is more
realistic and easier to create in colour, then create it in

*colour. Do whatever it is you want to do with this picture in order to make it as vivid as possible.*

### Stage Two
*Now you need to create an entirely different picture in your mind. This picture is a picture of yourself as you will be in the same circumstances when you have achieved your perfect weight and shape. Once again the picture can be in black and white or colour and be a snapshot or a film. Put as much effort into creating the most perfect scene as you possibly can, which will represent exactly how you will be and with all the most appealing features you will have, and what you will be doing when you have made the change. Make this picture as vivid as possible.*

### Stage Three
*This is where you switch one picture for another in your conscious and subconscious mind and this is how you do it.*

*First of all, make a large, vivid picture of the situation you feel most uncomfortable with as you did in Stage One. Next, in the bottom right-hand corner of this picture, make a small, dark version of the picture as you want to be and as you did in Stage Two.*

*Now you do the switch. Take the small picture and, in a fraction of a second, blow it up in size. Make it bright and vivid and see it in your mind bursting through the first picture and exploding on to the screen in your mind. As you do this and as the second picture bursts through the screen, say out loud and in a powerful voice, 'WOW', and hold that picture for five seconds.*

*Now open your eyes for a second, close them straight away and repeat the switch again. Do this again for a total of ten times and do not forget to open your eyes for a second between each one. Do these switches as quickly as you possibly can and every time the new picture bursts through the old picture, do not forget to say 'WOW' each time and with power.*

One repetition of these ten sets of PDP exercises is usually sufficient to overcome any resistance to acting as if you already are, even under the most difficult circumstances. If you feel the need to do this same exercise once or twice again over the next few days, you can of course do so.

You can also apply this same PDP exercise to numerous other situations where you may have difficulty in acting as if you already are, but having overcome the most difficult situation, it is unlikely that you will need to apply it to any other.

### How are you going to act now?

I said before that this is a very individual decision, but how about these for a few ideas to spark off your own imagination and remove a few more inhibitions?

Instead of taking a corner table in a restaurant or cafeteria, wearing a quiet dress or suit and sitting with your shoulders hunched, talking in a quiet voice, take a centre table where everyone can see you. Wear a bright and very noticeable outfit. Sit upright and talk animatedly and without self-consciousness.

If you drive a convertible car, and don't often take the hood down because you don't want to draw attention to yourself at the moment, but it is actually in your nature to be gregarious and outgoing, then take the hood down every day from now on. Put on a bright scarf, make yourself look good and feel good and go out and flaunt yourself for all you are worth.

Whatever it is that you would do when you have achieved your perfect weight and shape, act as if you already are. You will be amazed at the change in the way you feel and the effect that this has on you and on other people. It will also affect your body and the way it is able to help you achieve the weight and shape that you want to be. Act as if you are already what you want to be all day and every day from now on.

## WHAT SHOULD YOU EAT? YOUR BODY KNOWS BEST!

If you had lived hundreds of years ago and were not surrounded by hundreds of different, tempting, highly processed and denutrified foods, you would have no difficulty in selecting the most appropriate foods to eat. They would either have been fresh or rotten.

In today's world, apart from all the junk food, you also have a much wider choice of good, nutritious and delicious foods to eat than people ever had many years ago, and with only one exception, your body knows precisely what it should and should not be eating.

Your PDP exercises this week will include some techniques to get your subconscious mind back on track to select the right foods for you to be eating from now on. For those of you who need a little extra guidance on this subject, there is a seven-day eating plan in the appendix to help you in your choice of menus.

Please remember that this programme you are going through is a plan for life, not a six-week crash course, so – no replacement liquid meals, no fad diets and no fasting. These will do you no good whatsoever. Your body needs food, it knows what food is best and it knows how much it needs. Leave it to your subconscious mind and you will not ever have to worry about what to eat again.

## THE PRIMITIVE PROBLEM

I mentioned the exception to the 'your body knows best' rule and we should deal with this now. Your subconscious mind stores not only all the information that you have put into it over the years, but also some information that has been passed down from generation to generation. This is far more difficult to overcome and will require just a little conscious rather than subconscious effort on your part.

When man and woman first roamed the earth many thousands of years ago, food was scarce and the body, in conjunction with the subconscious mind, developed mechanisms to ensure the survival of the species. In particular, the body was guided to consume fat whenever possible and to conserve the fat by storing it in the body cells so that it could draw on these reserves in periods when there was no food available for consumption.

You probably already know that fat contains more calories than any other type of food, but you may not have been aware of the primitive connection. Knowledge is power, and therefore because you now know this, there is one thing that you must remember and be conscious of at all times. It is the simple fact that FAT makes FAT. So be aware of what you are eating, read your food labels and whenever and wherever it is possible to do so, avoid eating fat in any of its available forms.

There is of course a further problem associated with this primitive need for survival, and this is the body–mind connection.

The moment that your inner consciousness even so much as hears or senses the meaning of that word that I said we would not mention again, the body–mind response goes into action. The primitive part of your inner being instantly senses danger and alerts the chemical factory inside you of the potential danger it is facing. This causes your body to go into a defensive strategy and the primitive responses switch many of your cells into 'fat storage' mode. No matter how sensible you mean to be on your programme, the body wants to protect itself from you. It knows no better.

The key to avoiding your body taking this action against you and your plans to achieve your perfect weight and shape is of course Psycho-Dynamic Programming. The following exercise will allow you to teach your subconscious mind that, this time, it is all right to allow you to lose weight. It will learn to accept that this time, you are going to be sensible and will do it no harm whatsoever and that it's OK to cooperate with you instead of fight you. Try the following exercise now and use this every morning this week as part of your regular programme.

*Exercise:*
*Sit in a comfortable, upright chair and go through your breathing and relaxation exercises.*

*When you have completed this, I want you to visualise a picture of yourself sitting in this chair. See yourself sitting comfortably with your eyes closed, relaxed and calm. Hold that picture clearly for just a few seconds and then let the screen in front of your eyes go blank. You will see nothing but a dark screen. This is your subconscious mind.*

*Now visualise the following words printed clearly in large letters on that screen:*

*'It's all right for you to allow me to lose weight'*

*See those words clearly on the screen, hold the picture there in your mind and read those words over and over for the next ten minutes.*

## WHY DOES FAT ACCUMULATE IN CERTAIN PLACES?

Once again, this is a primitive function and there is a very logical answer to this question. There are certain cells in your body that tend to store fat more readily than others. These are sited in places where they are least likely to get in the way of other bodily functions and actions that you need to take throughout the day in order to function as a human being.

In most cases it is only when these particular sites are

full and overflowing that the body will start to try and find other sites to store fat. Most of these will be noticeable from the way that you look, although of course there are many internal parts of your body where fat can be stored and which can prove to be extremely dangerous. The arteries are one of the most well known of these and fatty deposits here can cause heart disease and heart failure.

Where are these sites? It is fairly obvious by now, is it not? Where are you currently storing your excess weight? Most people adopt one of two weight accumulation patterns. These are either the stomach, bottom, thighs and lower legs, or the stomach, chest, neck and upper and lower arms. If you are particularly overweight then you probably put additional supplies of fat in both of these areas. Very few people deviate very much from this pattern of weight accumulation.

Now I am going to teach you another exercise that you will use in conjunction with your PDP exercises this week and which will start to get rid of accumulated fat from the one area that will have more impact on your appearance than any other.

*Exercise:*
## RUB YOUR TUMMY AWAY IN TEN MINUTES A DAY

*If this seems a little ridiculous to you, I can assure you that it will not in a few days' time. I have taught hundreds of people this exercise and it has worked for every person that has taken it seriously. I once wrote an article for a national magazine describing this particular technique, and for months afterwards the magazine was deluged with letters and telephone calls from people wanting information on what else they could 'rub away'. So if you would like to rub your tummy away, this is what you should do.*

*Lie flat on the floor or on your bed and expose your stomach area. Keeping your eyes closed, hold your hand a very short distance from the surface of your skin, as close as possible, so that you can feel the heat from your hand against your skin and directly over your navel.*

*Now I want you to imagine the heat from your hand travelling down into your skin, going through the skin to the fat cells and I want you to see a picture in your mind of the fat cells dissolving and just melting away.*

*When you get this picture clearly into your mind, start to move your hand slowly in small circles and each time you complete a circle, make the next circle a tiny bit larger. All the time you are doing this, keep that clear picture in your mind of the heat travelling down from your hand and dissolving those accumulated fat cells.*

*Do this mental exercise every day for at least the next seven days at the end of your morning and evening PDP exercises. Seven days is all you will need to do this in order to set up the subconscious chain reaction that will melt the rest of your tummy away.*

## THE METABOLISM TEST

Before we go into your PDP exercise instructions for this week, there is one more thing that I would like you to do in order to give us both a gauge to the level of your metabolic rate and how quickly you put on or can take off weight.

Obtain a clinical thermometer calibrated in the Fahrenheit scale and every night for the next five nights, shake the thermometer down to well below normal before you go to bed. First thing in the morning, before you get up, go to the toilet, or in fact do anything, slip the thermometer under your tongue and leave it there for a few minutes. Record the temperature reading on the chart at the end of this chapter and I shall discuss the results of the test with you next week.

**Important Note:**
If you are female and menstruating, you must not start this test until twenty-four hours after your period has ceased. As far as this programme is concerned, it is perfectly all right if you have to wait until halfway through this week or even next week to carry out this test.

## YOUR PSYCHO-DYNAMIC PROGRAMMING EXERCISES FOR THIS WEEK

### Morning PDP Exercises

First of all, carry out your twenty-minute breathing and relaxation or pre-programming exercise. At the end of this period, carry out the exercise to programme your body that it is all right for you to lose weight. In addition to this, carry out the 'Rub Your Tummy Away' exercise.

### Evening PDP Exercises

Once again, go through the twenty-minute pre-programming exercises. When you have finished this stage, and for the next ten minutes, I want you to see yourself as if you were part of a film. Picture yourself exactly the perfect weight and shape you will be in the future and doing all the things that you have been doing this week as part of your 'acting as if you already are' exercises.

Picture yourself as you will be acting in the future. See yourself eating the right foods, exercising in a sensible and appropriate manner for your circumstances, and looking great, feeling good and interacting with your friends and acquaintances and enjoying life to the full. Picture yourself the 'star of your own show'.

Every time the picture you are seeing in your mind is one that is virtually perfect and is precisely how you want to be and are going to be, or whenever you are feeling really good about the picture and your body is feeling the experience with intensity, and whenever the sounds that *you hear and the internal dialogue are exciting you, make the picture even brighter in your mind and at the same time, touch the tip of your little finger and your thumb together and squeeze gently for three seconds. This will lock the picture into your subconscious mind.*

*In addition to this, spend an extra five minutes on the 'Rub Your Tummy Away' exercise.*

One last thing before you get on with this week's programme. I would just like to tell you one of my favourite sayings by one of my favourite authors, Richard Bach. This quote has always been a source of inspiration to me and I hope it will be to you.

> 'You are never given a wish without also being given the power to make it come true.'

Have a really good week!

## SUMMARY OF KEY POINTS

- Every conscious and subconscious thought you have creates a series of chemical reactions throughout your body. By changing your physical posture and facial expressions you can change what is going on in your subconscious and conscious mind. This is part of the power of PDP.
- Act as if you had already achieved your perfect weight and shape and enjoy yourself doing it.
- Your body knows what it should and should not eat. Trust it. The only exception to this is fat. Fat makes fat. Avoid all forms of fat in your food. If you need guidance on what constitutes sensible and nutritious eating habits, turn to the relevant section in the appendix.
- Carry out your morning and evening PDP exercises every day. At the end of these, carry out the 'Rub Your Tummy Away' exercise. If at the end of this you feel inclined to give your stomach muscles a little extra exercise, you may do so. Turn to the section in the appendix headed 'about exercise' for guidance.
- Carry out your metabolism test for five consecutive mornings as described and record the results on the progress monitor sheet.
- Complete your progress monitor sheet at the end of the week.

**PROGRESS MONITOR – PLEASE COMPLETE AT THE END OF THE LAST DAY OF THE WEEK**

**Instructions:**

Place a tick in the relevant column alongside each of the following questions. Do not think about your answers for too long – your initial reaction to each question will be the most accurate answer.

| Compared to when you first started this programme: | worse | the same | better | much better | very much better | totally satisfied |
|---|---|---|---|---|---|---|
| How do you feel about your weight and shape now? | | | | | | |
| How do you think other people feel about your weight and shape now? | | | | | | |
| How do you feel about yourself as a person, taking into account factors such as your confidence, personality, sense of humour and ability to relate to and communicate with other people? | | | | | | |
| If you are in a close relationship with another person, how do you feel about this relationship now? | | | | | | |
| If you are in a close relationship with another person, how do you think that other person feels about this relationship now? | | | | | | |
| How do you feel about your confidence and ability to achieve your perfect weight and shape in the future and keep it there for ever? | | | | | | |
| How do you feel about being able to eat less, and more sensibly and nutritiously, in the future? | | | | | | |
| How do you feel about your ability to maintain any form of general exercise routine in the future? | | | | | | |

My morning temperature readings were: Day 1    Day 2    Day 3    Day 4    Day 5

My average temperature was (add the above figures together and divide by 5):

# CHAPTER THREE

## WEEK THREE

# Be Positive – The Golden Key

Well, here we are at the beginning of Week Three of your programme. How are you feeling after the first two weeks? If my past experience of running these programmes is anything to go by, you are starting to feel very good about yourself. You still have some reservations about the techniques of Psycho-Dynamic Programming you are learning, but you also know that something very strange and powerful is happening to you and it is taking a little bit of getting used to. That is fine.

You are feeling better about the way you look, the way you feel and the way you relate to other people around you. Most important of all, you are starting to feel more positive about achieving your perfect weight and shape than you have ever felt before.

### A Gentle Reminder
Please remember that this programme was never intended to be a crash course for weight loss. You already knew that such programmes did not work before you even bought this book. The few people that do manage to lose

weight very quickly rarely manage to maintain this weight for very long and they usually look quite sick as a result of it.

People who undertake crash slimming programmes eat so little that they never have any energy for exercise. Even worse, they lose muscle and muscle tone instead of achieving fat loss; they lose more than a safe amount of water from their tissues and this dehydration is accompanied by a corresponding loss of essential vitamins and minerals. Crash slimming programmes can also cause a loss of essential protein and inflict immeasurable damage on the organs and tissues, and the loss of skin tone makes people undergoing these programmes look quite awful. Their bodies, and particularly their subconscious minds, go through the most terrible traumas. As a result of this, their bodies want to fight back to try and maintain their original status quo. As soon as their bodies have the strength and energy to do so, they pile the pounds back on as fast as they possibly can.

Our programme is very different. Ours is a gradual process where we re-educate the subconscious mind which in turn re-educates the body. The medium-term effects are just as dramatic as the short-term effects of any crash course, but they do you good instead of harm, and they will last indefinitely.

What you are putting into your subconscious mind now and over the next few weeks will teach it all that it will ever need to know to enable you to attain your ideal weight, look better and feel better. It will give you the energy, vigour, creativity and positive attitude that will enable you to enjoy life to its fullest extent.

## BEING POSITIVE IS A KEY FACTOR

Let us focus on that word 'positive' for a while, because being positive is a key ingredient in this programme, not only in relation to your weight and shape but also to everything else that happens to you on your journey through life. It can mean the difference between spending your three score years and ten, and hopefully more, enjoying everything that life has to offer and making whatever you want happen for you, or being a victim to circumstances and letting life lead you through all the trials and tribulations that it can have in store for those who choose to allow it to heap problems upon them.

Take a look around you and think of all the very successful and positive people that you know and possibly admire. How many of these people are really overweight? You may know a few, but those that are have normally chosen to be so and are happy with their weight and shape.

Positive people move fast. And when they move fast, their subconscious moves fast as well. When that starts to happen, you now know that everything else in the body starts to move more quickly too. Positive people do not have the time to put on weight; their minds and their bodies are too busy looking for the next challenge, the new excitement and the stimulation to get more and more out of their lives. That does not mean that they are always on the move, of course.

Positive people also know how to relax and get more enjoyment out of their relaxation time than those who are less positive. The difference is that whilst they are enjoying their relaxation time, their subconscious minds are programmed to maintain their cellular structure and weight stabilisation systems so that they do not go into an immediate slump and start to put on weight.

## THE METABOLIC TEST RESULTS

Before we go any further on the subject of being positive, let us take a look at your morning temperature readings and what they could mean. If you were unable to complete these tests last week, remember to re-read this and the following page next week.

The 'normal' temperature range is between 97.8 degrees Fahrenheit and 98.4 degrees Fahrenheit. If your average temperature over the five-day test period was 97.4 degrees or less, then you probably have a slightly lower than normal metabolic rate. Do not start to worry about this. You almost certainly do not have a medical condition that requires any form of treatment whatsoever. If you did, you would be experiencing many other unpleasant symptoms as well. You just happen to be running a little slower than some other people, and in my experience, over eighty per cent of my overweight patients had exactly the same condition.

This condition and what it causes is not dissimilar to what happens with the engine in your car if it is not idling at the right speed. In this condition, and when it is stationary, it is not keeping all the parts properly coated in oil. Particles of carbon accumulate in corners of the engine and other areas where they should not and the whole system starts to clog up. It becomes a little bit more difficult to get started in the morning and even when it is running, a sudden push on the accelerator pedal can cause it to stall.

A similar situation is happening inside your body and, just like the car engine, all it needs is a few simple adjustments to set the idling speed correctly. This condition is so common that I expect a very high proportion of readers to exhibit the same temperature results.

What can you do about this? Well, apart from the fact that being more positive can help to speed up your body and therefore your ability to lose weight, there are also some PDP exercises that can assist, and you will carry these out after your morning breathing and relaxation exercises. Some additional nutritional support may also be required, so turn to the relevant section in the appendix for this information.

If you are one of the readers who were in the normal temperature range, you will be instructed on an alternative morning PDP exercise.

## HOW CAN YOU BECOME MORE POSITIVE?

You need something else to do in your life apart from what you are already doing – just one more thing that excites you, that will fit into your available time or that you can fit in with a little reshuffling of your present arrangements. And I don't want to hear that you are too busy. Yes, I know that you are going to have to find just a little time every day for some exercise on top of the extra hour that you need for your PDP exercise, but so what?

Have you ever heard the expression, 'If you want something done, ask a busy person to do it for you'? The sort of busy person referred to here is someone who is positive, busy and yet can always find a little extra time to do something that they would like to do. That something could be helping a friend out with something that the friend is too busy to do, helping the kids with their homework, joining a committee, a new challenge they feel like taking on in their lives or whatever else is asked of them or they choose to do.

## DEFINING YOUR GOALS

If you have a job and feel you could be doing more and contributing more, then plan how to do it. Maybe you are looking for a promotion, more money and more job satisfaction? Maybe in the longer term you want the boss's job? Or maybe you are currently out of work and looking for a new job or career to pursue. Then again, you may be running your own business and have much greater potential than you are currently achieving.

Whatever it is that you want can be yours using the techniques of Psycho-Dynamic Programming. The first step is to define precisely what you want to happen!

You may be wondering why I want you to do something else in addition to achieving your ideal weight and shape. Well, in the first place, I am really not taking up very much of your time and I would like to divert your conscious mind from making this programme its focal point over the coming weeks. Your subconscious mind is going to take care of your weight and shape. Secondly, I want you to prove to yourself that you can get really positive and have fun doing something else or improving something else in your life.

So what would you like to do?

## Julie's Story

Julie was a very young forty-five-year-old woman who had got married at an early age and whose children were now grown up and had flown the nest. Julie's husband had a good job and they had no financial worries at all. Her relationship with her husband seemed to be 'normal' for a couple who had been together for over twenty years. Julie came to see me because she was putting on weight and her eating habits were getting very much out of control.

It soon became very obvious that Julie was eating out of pure frustration. She felt that she wanted to do something with her life that was more positive than just socialising with her friends for most of the day, but she just could not identify what it was that she wanted to do, and this was causing her to eat her way into an even bigger problem.

I knew that if Julie could just find the solution, her eating problem could be dealt with very easily. I also knew that if she did not find the answer, then her eating problem was rapidly going to become far more serious than it was at the time.

The first thing that I explained to Julie was that what she was having was not a problem but an opportunity crisis. Let's face it, how many of us are free of financial worries, have a fairly good relationship with their partners and have the time and opportunity to make a new life plan?

This is what I asked Julie to do. You should do the same.

*Exercise:*
*Go to a favourite place in your home, somewhere where*
*you feel safe and secure and where you are not going to be*
*disturbed for the next hour or so. Take several sheets of*
*writing paper and a pen and sit down comfortably in your*
*favourite chair.*

*Now I want you to imagine that there are absolutely no*
*limitations to what you can achieve as a person and that*
*whatever you decide to do, your success is absolutely*
*guaranteed.*

*I want you to get totally into that frame of mind and start*
*writing a list and keep writing for at least twenty minutes.*
*Let your mind roam totally free and think in Auditory,*
*Visual and Kinaesthetic modes. Hear the words in your*
*head, see pictures of what it is you can do and experience*
*the feelings, the smell and the touch of these achievements.*

*When you write your list, be very careful not to use any*
*negative expressions. The word 'try', for example, is a*
*'no-no'! Each item on your list should begin with 'I can' or*
*'I will'. Start making your list now.*

*When you have finished the first part of this exercise, take*
*a fresh sheet of paper and decide how long the project*
*should take to give you the greatest possible personal*
*satisfaction. Remember it is your satisfaction that we are*
*talking about here, so how your project might affect*
*someone else is irrelevant. Will you be happier if you have*
*achieved something in one month, three months, six*

*months, or will your greatest satisfaction come from working on a longer term goal? Make that decision now.*

*Next, based on your most satisfactory time frame, go back over the first list and cross out every item that does not fit into this time frame. Then, from the remaining list, select one and at the most two items that you most want to achieve.*

Julie came up with the following:
    1 – 'I will become a garden designer.'
    2 – 'I will have a better relationship with my partner.'

What was the most important item on your list?

I will not discuss with you how we dealt with the second item on Julie's list; I shall save that for next week, as it may have some relevance to your own situation.

As for Julie's first item and your own, these are the next steps.

*Exercise:*
## DEFINE YOUR STRATEGY TO ACHIEVE THIS GOAL

*Without a definite strategy you cannot achieve your goal. A goal without a strategy is like a map with all the details missing. Just a meaningless overview. A map with all the routes and towns marked clearly upon it enables you to plan your route with minute detail and guarantee your safe arrival. So it is with your life plan when you have the strategy in place. When you have laid down a detailed strategy for getting from A to B, each step of the way, the chances of your arriving at your destination are down to judgement, not luck.*

*What do you need to put a strategy together to accomplish your goal? Think of a time in your life when you were totally successful at achieving something that you set out to do. What did you have to do to achieve this? Which of your strengths did you use, which of your talents? Write them down.*

*Now relate that experience to your new goal and write down your strategy to achieve this based on your previous success. What will you have to do each step of the way? Whose help might you need and what resources, if any, will you need to accomplish this?*

*When you have written down your action plan, spend a little time experiencing how you will feel when you have achieved this. Hear, see and feel the success that you are going to achieve. Enjoy this experience for all it is worth.*

*What is the first step you need to take and what can you do today to put this plan into action? Decide on that first step now and do it now. Making that first step is a little like firing an arrow at a target. You can take all the time that you like to draw back the bowstring and take aim. You can even put down the bow and arrow and pick them up again later. But once the arrow has been released and is on its way, nothing can stop it!*

*Your PDP exercises this week will also help you to achieve this new dimension in your life.*

## SUBCONSCIOUS MIND TRIGGERS
Being positive is just so important that in addition to your PDP exercises this week, I want you to be able to give your subconscious mind a series of constant jogs and reminders throughout the day. Here is how you can achieve this.

*Exercise:*
Go out and purchase a pack of very small self-adhesive labels. You will need about fifty of these altogether. Twenty-five will be required for this exercise and you will need another twenty-five for later on in the programme. These need be no bigger than about five millimetres across, but any size will do. If you can get them in your two most favourite colours, even better.

When you have acquired these labels, I want you to put a small cross on each one of them indicating a 'positive sign'. I then want you to stick these labels in various places so that you will come across them constantly throughout the day. You can fix one on the face of your watch, the rear-view mirror of your car and the speedometer, your briefcase, your time planner, your favourite mug, the refrigerator door and your bathroom mirror. Affix them to the surfaces that are likely to catch your eye most frequently.

After a time you will not notice these labels with your conscious mind but your subconscious mind will be picking up the message and constantly reinforcing your more positive attitude.

## EXERCISE AND YOUR AIM TO ACHIEVE YOUR PERFECT WEIGHT AND SHAPE

Exercise is an essential part of almost every weight loss programme. If you have chosen to achieve a dramatic change in your weight and shape, then this one is no different. However, you will be very surprised at just how little exercise you really need in order to achieve your perfect weight and shape.

Why is some exercise so important? There have been numerous studies on this subject and some of the findings may surprise you.

First of all, any type of aerobic exercise reduces the appetite. You will want to eat less, not more, and that has to be a good thing. Any form of aerobic exercise will do, and you will need to set aside fifteen minutes every day for this if you are not doing it already. Fifteen minutes is hardly any time at all.

The definition of aerobic exercise is any form of exercise which increases your heart rate and moves more oxygen around your cardiovascular system. In order to ensure that you are exercising aerobically, you just need to check your pulse rate from time to time. The pulse rate should be 180 beats per minute minus your age. If you have any form of medical condition which you believe may be aggravated by aerobic exercise, speak to your medical practitioner before embarking on this part of the programme. If they advise against anything other than a fairly brisk walk, this will do fine.

There are various forms of aerobic exercise that you can consider. Jogging is certainly not a favourite of everyone but if it suits you, that is great. You can also cycle, either using a regular bicycle or a stationary exercise model. You can always use the latter whilst watching a TV programme or listening to the radio. It is amazing how quickly fifteen minutes goes by. You can swim, trampoline, join in an aerobic exercise class, or any other form of exercise that raises your pulse rate to the required level. I even know of one of our patients who used to stop the newspaper delivery boy at the beginning of her street every morning and deliver the newspapers for him. That very brisk twenty-minute delivery round turned out to be one of the highlights of her day. In addition to that, the newspaper boy bought her a Christmas present.

There is another form of exercise that you may need to consider if your shape is a consideration. This is spot-reducing exercises, which are described in the appendix. Spot-reducing exercises will help you firm and tone the muscles in particular areas of your body and will give you a huge boost by improving your shape more rapidly.

I do not want you to rush into any exercise programme that you are not currently doing and enjoying. By carrying out your PDP exercises this week, you will find that by the end of the week you will have subconsciously decided what is the most suitable and enjoyable form of exercise for you and your subconscious mind will be programmed to make you want to do this without any effort or willpower being required. So please, no dashing off to the gym with your best friend this afternoon if you have never been there before. If you do, it is most unlikely that you will keep to a routine. Just be relaxed about the thought of exercising and wait and see what your subconscious mind comes up with for you later in the week.

## YOUR PSYCHO-DYNAMIC PROGRAMMING EXERCISES FOR THIS WEEK

### Morning PDP Exercises

First of all, carry out your twenty-minute relaxation and pre-programming exercise. At the end of this period, use PDP One if your average temperature on your metabolic test was 97.4 degrees Fahrenheit or less. If it was higher, then use PDP Two.

### PDP One

At the end of your pre-programming exercise, keeping your eyes closed, repeat the following statement silently to yourself and keep repeating this for a full ten minutes:

*'I (your name) am achieving my perfect weight. My body knows what it needs to do to assist me and those slower parts are speeding up to make me achieve my perfect shape. My body is working faster to make me achieve this and anything else I wish in the most sensible period of time.'*

### PDP Two

At the end of your pre-programming exercise, keeping your eyes closed, repeat the following statement silently to yourself and keep repeating this for a full ten minutes.

*'I (your name) am achieving my perfect weight and shape. My body and my mind are so positive and can make me achieve this and anything else I wish to achieve in the most sensible period of time.'*

*In addition to these exercises, spend an extra five minutes on the 'Rub Your Tummy Away' exercise.*

*Evening PDP Exercises*
*Once again, go through the pre-programming exercise. At the end of this twenty minutes, I want you to select the part of the body which you most want to improve the shape of. If this is a part of the body that you can comfortably reach, then place your hands upon the muscles there and squeeze and release them with your hands whilst tensing and relaxing the muscles. If you cannot reach them or cannot tense and relax them, do one or the other.*

*While you are doing this, I want you to let your mind wander to a time when you most enjoyed some form of exercise and remember what it was associated with. If it was a walk through a forest in early spring, picture that walk in your mind. Remember how you felt and remember the sounds that you heard. All the time continue squeezing and releasing those muscles. Perhaps it was a time when you used to exercise in a gymnasium or attend a dance or yoga class. Perhaps it was a sport that you made time for a long while ago. Whatever it is that you can remember that is associated with any type of exercise, picture this vividly in your mind and re-experience everything about it whilst squeezing and releasing those muscles.*

*Whenever you feel that experience at its peak moments, remember to touch the tip of your little finger and thumb together and squeeze gently. This will help to lock that experience into your subconscious mind.*

*Do this exercise for a full ten minutes.*

## SUMMARY OF KEY POINTS

- This is not a crash course in losing weight – they do not work! You are going to achieve your perfect weight and shape and maintain it indefinitely. This will take only a little longer.

- If you were menstruating last week, carry out the metabolic test described in week two for five consecutive mornings this week and enter the results on your progress monitor chart.

- Slim people are positive people. Become positive about doing something extra in your life, no matter how small or insignificant or how dramatic and impossible it might seem at first.

- Define what it is you want to achieve, define your strategy for achieving it and take the first step now.

- Acquire a quantity of self-adhesive labels in your favourite colour and put a cross on each one. Affix them in places where you will come across them frequently throughout the day.

- Exercise is an essential part of any weight loss and maintenance programme. By the end of this week your subconscious mind will have decided the most sensible and enjoyable form of exercise for you and will be programmed to make you want to do this. You will just ease yourself into it gently and will require no will-power to maintain the programme.

- If you wish to improve your shape more rapidly, turn to the spot-reducing exercises in the appendix.

- Carry out your morning and evening pre-programming exercises and, depending upon the results of your metabolic test, select the appropriate PDP exercise for the morning session.

- Complete your progress monitor chart at the end of the week.

PROGRESS MONITOR – PLEASE COMPLETE AT THE END OF THE LAST DAY OF THE WEEK

**Instructions:**

Place a tick in the relevant column alongside each of the following questions. Do not think about your answers for too long – your initial reaction to each question will be the most accurate answer.

| Compared to when you first started this programme: | worse | the same | better | much better | very much better | totally satisfied |
|---|---|---|---|---|---|---|
| How do you feel about your weight and shape now? | | | | | | |
| How do you think other people feel about your weight and shape now? | | | | | | |
| How do you feel about yourself as a person, taking into account factors such as your confidence, personality, sense of humour and ability to relate to and communicate with other people? | | | | | | |
| If you are in a close relationship with another person, how do you feel about this relationship now? | | | | | | |
| If you are in a close relationship with another person, how do you think that other person feels about this relationship now? | | | | | | |
| How do you feel about your confidence and ability to achieve your perfect weight and shape in the future and keep it there for ever? | | | | | | |
| How do you feel about being able to eat less, and more sensibly and nutritiously, in the future? | | | | | | |
| How do you feel about your ability to maintain any form of general exercise routine in the future? | | | | | | |

Complete if you were not able to carry out the Metabolic Test last week.

My morning temperature readings were: Day 1    Day 2    Day 3    Day 4    Day 5

My average temperature was (add the above figures together and divide by 5):

# CHAPTER FOUR

## WEEK FOUR

# How You Feel is How You Look

**IT'S YOUR RESPONSIBILITY**

There is absolutely nothing that can affect the way you look more than the way you feel. Some of the most stunning women I have ever met have been overweight by most people's standards, but because they were successful in their own minds and felt great about themselves, they looked great, and everyone ignored their size and envied their personalities and joy for life.

By contrast, I have also known many famous women who had what many would believe to be the most perfect figures but whose lives were miserable in spite of how most people perceived them on stage or screen. The way they felt and acted when not in the public's view was a far cry from their screen image. Without the expert attention of the make-up artists and the director's instructions on how to stand and force a smile for the cameras or their fans, the real image they presented left very little to envy.

How you feel emotionally is how you look physically. When you are feeling down, your posture slumps, the muscles in your face lose their natural tightness, your skin loses its natural sheen and healthy radiance and you look as awful as you feel.

However you do feel, let me make it perfectly clear to you, it is your responsibility, not some other person's. That may seem like a tough statement to make and a little unbelievable at first, but let me illustrate the proof of this by telling you a little story that I often tell people when they find this as hard to accept as I suspect you may do.

One day a woman walked into a doctor's waiting room. She was depressed and feeling bad-tempered, and the occupants in the waiting room gave her the perfect opportunity to vent her pent-up venom.

Sitting quietly, waiting for their turn to see the doctor, were three bald and bespectacled men. Seating herself opposite them, she said in a loud voice, 'I think all bald men who wear glasses look stupid!'

The reaction from each of these gentlemen was very different.

The first man became very red in the face, very angry, and, shaking his fist at the woman, uttered an extremely rude and unflattering retort.

The second of the three men took completely the opposite view. He burst out laughing at what he thought was the woman's stupidity. He was not in the least bothered by her statement and in fact it amused him considerably.

The third man sat absolutely still and silent. His expression changed not one bit. It was almost as if he had not heard what she had said. However, I can tell you that the following day, he felt so humiliated and concerned by her outburst that he went to the optician and ordered contact lenses, then to a gentleman's hairdressers, where he bought himself a wig.

So there you have it. One statement and yet each one of those men chose to react totally differently. They chose how they felt.

Those of you who are a little familiar with psycho-therapy, and many practitioners in that profession, might choose to lay the blame for these differing reactions on some deep-rooted event or series of events experienced in early childhood. That might be the case, but it does not alter the fact that the person still made the choice. It is their subconscious minds that they have to live with for the rest of their lives, and life is not a rehearsal – it is the real thing. If you can accept that how you feel is your responsibility and choose to do something about it, then you can only feel better and look better as a result.

Before we take a closer look at what you are choosing to feel about your life at the moment, I want to go into just a little detail on the way food can affect you and how you feel, and how the right choice of foods can make you feel better and look better and help you achieve your ideal weight and shape.

## NATURAL UPPERS AND DOWNERS – THE NUTRIENT CONNECTION

It is not my intention to deluge you with a mass of technical information, and I certainly do not want to turn you into a 'food faddie', but there are some basic things that you need to know about the foods that you eat in order for you to benefit from the sustained lift to your physical and mental well-being that certain foods can provide.

There are also certain types of foods that rob your body of valuable nutrients and will naturally depress you, and other foods that, whilst they have no effect on many people, can cause a reaction in others that makes them artificially depressed and can even cause them to eat much more of that same food in the mistaken belief that it is making them feel better. Hence the vicious cycle of binge eating. Like the 'Primitive Problem', this is an example of the body not knowing what is best for it.

If you want to know more detailed information about nutrition, there are many excellent books on the market, some of which are mentioned in the appendix. I am going to concentrate entirely on providing you with sufficient information to help you in your aim to achieve your perfect weight and shape in the shortest possible time and with the simplest explanation. I shall also help you to identify if there are any particular foods that may be causing you a problem.

## THE MAIN FOOD GROUPS
There are basically three main food groups. These are fats, proteins and carbohydrates. Apart from a varying degree of pleasure that people get from eating certain types of foods, the actual purpose of eating is to provide the body with essential nutrients contained within these foods which help to make it work properly. These nutrients

help to rebuild and replace cells that naturally die after they have served their purpose in keeping you alive and well and to provide energy for the cells to function properly in order for you to go about your life in the most enjoyable way.

## Fats

Fats are easily recognisable to most people. They contain more calories than most other foods, take longer to digest and break down into their component parts, and are the type of foods that are most easily stored by the body as fat when they are not needed for energy and other essential processes that take place in the body.

A certain amount of fat is essential for your natural health and well-being. However, no matter how careful you are in trying to avoid it, it is almost impossible not to consume more fat in your food than is necessary for your good health. Fats are hidden in very small amounts in so many foods that you would not find it possible to avoid them altogether and therefore my previous instructions stand. Avoid fat as much as you possibly can. Fat Makes Fat!

## Proteins

Proteins contain all sorts of good things for the body. Once the essential nutrients have been removed by your digestive juices and sent to where they are going to be used most effectively by the body, the rest of the protein is broken down into substances that help to replace the cells that have died and need replacing. These substances are called amino acids.

On the bad side of the protein coin, the waste products of protein digestion can be very poisonous if kept in the body for too long and can slow down many other processes within the body. Bearing in mind that we want your body to work quickly and efficiently to get you to your perfect weight and shape as soon as possible, it is essential that you eat the type of protein that contains the least amount of poisons and whose waste products can be expelled most effectively.

Proteins are found in meat, fish, eggs, vegetables, salads and all types of cereals and grains. As a simple rule of thumb, the heavier and denser the protein is in its original state, before preparation for eating, the worse it is likely to be for you. I emphasise, food preparation can often disguise the real culprits. As an example, take meat.

Whilst I am not suggesting you avoid meat altogether, it is one of the heaviest and densest proteins, one of the most difficult to digest and one which produces the largest amount of poisons. It should therefore be restricted in your diet. A large, juicy steak is easy to spot as a potential hazard when eaten in quantity, but when it is ground up and prepared to be served as a hamburger or pâté, its texture and consistency can be misleading. Whenever you are not sure about what type of protein to eat, think about it in its original state and you will not go far wrong.

I am sure that you have seen travel documentaries and similar programmes on the television, and in particular you may have seen films of tribes in Africa, Ethiopia and other far-flung places where people live on almost nothing but grains and cereals. There are very few, if any, fat people in these tribes. They are almost always slim, strong, sinewy, well-shaped and graceful. Much of this is due to the fact that they eat little or no meat and get an awful lot of natural exercise.

A little of what you fancy almost always does you good and so do please enjoy that juicy steak or other meat that you eat from time to time. Just do not overdo it. Remember that meat in anything other than moderate quantities is the least essential and most damaging ingredient after fat in your quest to achieve your perfect weight and shape. All of the other types of protein mentioned above will serve your purpose much better, particularly if you eat them in slightly lesser quantities than you have in the past.

## Carbohydrates

The last main food group is carbohydrates. Essentially, carbohydrates are broken down into sugar in the body. Some carbohydrates are broken down quickly and are called simple carbohydrates. Others take longer to digest and are called complex carbohydrates. Apart from the fact that you know that too much sugar will make you fat, whatever form you take it in, there are some people who need to be concerned about eating carbohydrates for other, more serious reasons. I shall cover this point shortly.

The main food sources of sugars and carbohydrates are fairly obvious, particularly simple sugars. Simple sugars are simply that, sweet things that either occur naturally or are processed to make them sweeter and more attractive to eat. It is not difficult to spot white sugar or brown sugar on its own, but it is a little more difficult to recognise other sugars such as sucrose, glucose or fructose when they are combined with other food. So read the ingredients labels when buying anything in a jar, tube, can or packet.

Simple sugars taste sweet and if you have a sweet tooth, you are likely to have the problem I mentioned above. Simple sugars are digested too quickly by the body, which cannot utilise the energy that is produced as quickly as it is produced and therefore stores it in your body. Simple sugars make you fat!

Complex carbohydrates are mainly found in cereals and grains, vegetables and fruits, but there are a lot of other sources as well. The less carbohydrates have been altered during processing, the better they are likely to be for you in reducing and controlling your weight. If you want to feel fuller for longer and want to eat less and feel fuller, then unprocessed carbohydrates are better for you: brown rice instead of white rice, brown bread instead of white bread and wholemeal pasta instead of white pasta. Choices like this can make some considerable difference to the rate at which you achieve your perfect weight.

Complex carbohydrates are good for most people. They make you feel full, they take longer for the body to digest, they can give you a long-lasting source of energy and can be an essential source of vitamins and minerals. However, for some people, they can be a major problem.

## CARBOHYDRATE INTOLERANCE

The subject of carbohydrate intolerance, or carbohydrate allergy as it is sometimes called, is almost as complex as the molecular structure of a complex carbohydrate, and it took me quite a while to redefine the information into a quick and easy guide for you.

Carbohydrate intolerance can cause food addictions and binge eating and this can sometimes lead to bulimia and anorexia nervosa. As you know, these are two terrible conditions. Carbohydrate intolerance can also cause mood swings, depression, and unnatural highs which automatically lead to unnatural lows and can make you tense, irritable and unsociable.

Carbohydrate intolerance can make you fat because of these mind-altering effects and can also make you fat because of the effect it has on your internal organs.

Much of how your body works and deals with food has to do with many of the organs and glands in your body. The thyroid gland is a perfect example, and I am sure that most people are aware that an underactive thyroid can cause you to gain a lot of unnecessary weight. The same is true for many other glands in your body. If you have an intolerance or allergy to carbohydrates in either the simple or complex form, you will put on a lot of extra weight and find it hard to get rid of it until you remove the offending foods from your diet. As you can see, it is a complex problem.

Carbohydrate intolerance is a particularly difficult problem for three reasons. In the first place, you are unlikely to be intolerant to all forms of carbohydrate. Secondly, carbohydrates are not always easy to spot in your diet. The following foods all contain carbohydrates:

| | | |
|---|---|---|
| Orange Juice | Cornflakes | Skimmed milk |
| Sugar | Hamburgers | Yoghurt |
| Coleslaw | Diet Pepsi | Tonic Water |
| French Fries | Tomato Soup | Baked Potatoes |
| Peas | Melons | Bananas |

You can see from the above very short list that it is not quite as obvious as you might first think which foods contain carbohydrates.

Thirdly, and far more importantly from the point of view of achieving your perfect weight and shape, this is another case where the body does not know what is best. In fact the opposite is true: the body actually craves more of that very same food that it is intolerant or allergic to, and the moment it has experienced a little of it, it wants a lot more. Fortunately for you, if you are one of the many people who are carbohydrate intolerant, it is that last statement that is also the clue to spotting and dealing with the problem and most other food allergy problems.

## How to spot if you are carbohydrate intolerant

*Exercise:*
*Can you answer yes to any of the following statements?*

*I often feel very low and use sweets and chocolates as an instant pick-me-up. When I do, I eat a lot and very quickly, almost without tasting them.*

*I crave certain types of foods much more than others.*

*If I am feeling low, certain types of foods give me an immediate and almost abnormal lift.*

*When I am alone and even if I am not hungry, I tend to look for and eat a particular type of food.*

*When I am shopping with a list, I often buy a particular item or items of food on impulse, particularly those that give me an instant craving when I see them.*

*When I eat, there are certain foods that I gobble down very quickly, almost without chewing or tasting them.*

*When I eat, there are certain types of food that always make me crave second or even third helpings.*

*There are some foods that make me feel very tired after I have eaten them.*

If you have answered yes to more than three of the above questions, you almost certainly have an intolerance to some carbohydrates. If you have answered yes to nearly all those questions, you are probably allergic to many if not all carbohydrates.

So what can you do about it?

The simplest solution is to be aware. Because of the PDP exercises that you have been doing for the last few weeks, you are already much more aware of your body anyway, and it should be a simple matter to focus on the above questions and notice how you and your body react in different circumstances.

If you crave a certain type of food much more than any other type of food, avoid it. Remember that you have a choice, not only in how you feel and how you look but also in what you eat. If you want to look good and feel good, then decide to choose wisely. If there is any food that definitely fulfils the criteria laid down above, then do your very best to avoid eating it. If you have answered yes to most or all of the above questions and believe that you have a very high intolerance to carbohydrates, then I suggest you consult a physician who specialises in nutritional therapy.

## VITAMINS AND MINERALS

Vitamins and minerals are essential nutrients that are found in almost all foods to a greater or lesser extent. The more processed foods are, the less likely they are to contain adequate quantities of these nutrients and the more likely you are to feel unwell. If you feel unwell, then you look unwell. Moreover, if you are unwell, then your body will find it more difficult to lose weight as effectively as it might otherwise. In addition to that, a lack of certain vital nutrients can cause a variety of physical and emotional problems which can have a negative effect on this programme.

Many doctors will tell you that supplementing your diet with nutritional supplements is unwise and unnecessary. I violently disagree. The way foods are commercially farmed nowadays, they do not contain the amounts of these essential nutrients that are found in organically grown foods grown in naturally enriched soils. In my opinion, supplementation of the diet with extra supplies of these nutrients is essential.

Once again, I do not intend to go into too much detail on the role of vitamins and minerals in maintaining health and am not dealing with them in this chapter. If you have any of the problems listed below, all of which can have a negative physical and emotional effect on your aim to achieve your perfect weight and shape, then turn to the relevant section in the appendix where I deal with the nutritional support of these conditions. If you want to learn more about nutritional therapy there are many excellent books on the market and some of these are listed in the appendix. You could also consult an appropriately qualified expert in this field and the relevant section in the appendix will help you to find one.

Turn to the appendix for nutritional support if:

- Your metabolism test showed an average of 97.4 degrees Fahrenheit or less.

- You have any skin or hair problems that prevent you from looking and therefore feeling your best.
- You are underweight and are having difficulty putting on weight.
- You feel particularly stressed or depressed.
- You have low energy levels and are feeling tired.
- You suffer from constipation or diarrhoea.

## PSYCHO-SLIMMING TIPS – SOME HELPFUL EATING HABITS

Before I go on to discuss some of the other ways you can feel better about yourself, and some of the things that might be getting in the way, here are just a few simple and common-sense tips that can work miracles if you have decided to eat less.

### Psycho-Slimming Tip One
*When you are eating, concentrate!*
Your subconscious mind is very much in control of a lot of your habits by now, but it cannot help you to control how much you are eating by itself just yet.

Your appetite is switched off by a hormone in the brain and your brain does not switch off this hormone when you have had enough to eat. This hormone is only released when it is *told* that you have had enough. So for the next few weeks and until your subconscious mind is totally in control, no watching television, no listening to the radio and no reading your newspaper, magazine, this book or any other book while you are eating. Concentrate on what you are eating, enjoy it, and tell your body when you know you have had enough.

**Psycho-Slimming Tip Two**
*Enjoy your food*
Eating can be a lot of fun and a much greater pleasure than most people believe. When you are eating, chew your food slowly. Savour the taste and the smell and the texture of the food. When you eat slowly and enjoy it, you will be very pleasantly surprised at just how little you need to be satisfied and full.

**Psycho-Slimming Tip Three**
*Use a smaller plate than you usually do!*
A large amount of food on a very large plate still does not look very much. By contrast, a moderate amount of good food on a small plate can look an awful lot more. You can also use a much smaller knife, fork and spoon than you usually do. This will have the same effect. You could even take to using chopsticks. Apart from a few Sumo wrestlers, I know of very few overweight Japanese or Chinese people.

**Psycho-Slimming Tip Four**
*You do not have to clean your plate!*
Of course it is wasteful and wicked to waste food, and when you are in control of the situation you should not cook more than you know is the right amount for you to eat. When you are not in control, it is not your fault if you are given more than you need and want. Do not clean the plate because food is left upon it. Stop eating when you have had enough.

**Psycho-Slimming Tip Five**
*The Fingertip Technique!*
During your PDP exercises over the last few weeks, at those moments when you have been experiencing your most exciting and emotional experiences, you have been locking these experiences into your subconscious mind by touching the tip of your little finger against the tip of your thumb and pressing them gently but firmly against each other. If, at any time during the programme, you feel the need for a little extra help from your subconscious mind, simply repeat that exercise. All the power that you have locked into your subconscious mind is available to you instantly when you do this.

## YOUR PROGRESS TO DATE
Let us have a quick review of where you are so far on this programme. Take a look at your Progress Monitor chart that you completed at the end of last week. I am quite certain that you will agree with the following points.

- You have decided what your perfect weight and shape should be.
- You already feel more comfortable with your weight and shape and you are very confident that you are going to achieve the results that you want.
- You feel better about eating less, and more sensibly, and you are slowly but surely becoming accustomed to the thought that you are establishing an exercise routine that is really going to work for you and is one that you can and will maintain for life.

- You feel better about yourself than you have for a long time. You are becoming more and more positive about yourself and most other people are feeling better about you too.

## YOUR CLOSEST RELATIONSHIP – MANAGING CHANGE

What about the current partner in your life? How are they feeling about you and how are you feeling about them? Does this part of your life lack the level of improvement that you have achieved in all those other areas? Perhaps it is even a little worse?

Change of any sort is unnerving for most people, and most will try to resist it at almost any cost. Any disruption to their normal pattern of life, whether for better or for worse, can cause worry, restlessness and unease. When the change is one that is out of their control, it can give rise to panic and paranoia. When someone close to them is changing, and that is out of their control, it can cause the most devastating feelings imaginable. Fear of change is basic to human nature.

You have now learned to take responsibility for your own feelings and actions and know that you can choose how you want to feel. Your partner may not know that they can choose how to feel about your changing, and even if they do, they may be choosing to fight and resist it simply because they are scared of the change and how it might affect them.

If the partner you are with is the person that you wanted to be with when you started this relationship and is the person that you still want to be with, then you owe it to yourself to choose to take responsibility for healing the situation. This will mean improving how they feel about you and how you feel about them. When you have achieved this, you will feel so much better about yourself, look so much better and will have the support and encouragement that will guarantee that one of the last few remaining obstacles to achieving your perfect weight has been removed.

## Take a short cut and then work backwards

Do you remember Julie from last week? Julie's second aim was to improve her relationship with her partner. Just as she had been able to come to a decision on her other priority so quickly and achieve immediate results, she wanted to apply the same sense of urgency to her personal relationship and was excited at the thought.

For this week I would like you also to consider taking a short cut. We will be dealing with relationships next week and in some considerable detail. In the meantime if, like Julie, you want some immediate and dramatic results and you are prepared to take the responsibility for achieving them, there is no better time to start than right now.

Any type of relationship can be improved. Like Julie, it can be the relationship you have with your partner. It could also be the relationship you have with your best friend or any other friend. It can also be relationships that you have at work, socially or just with people in general. Whichever of your relationships you are least satisfied with, improving them will also have a dramatic effect on improving your weight and shape.

## PSYCHO-RELATIVE THERAPY

There are so many different facets to any one individual, many of them changing constantly as that individual reacts to their environment and the people around them. Put two individuals together in a relationship and you have the most complex subject in all of the world to deal with. I could write a book on this subject alone and in fact intend to do so. In the meantime, in the space of a few pages, I need to introduce you to a few simple concepts and a PDP exercise that, together, will make a major difference to your understanding of yourself and your relationships with other people. They will also affect the way you feel about yourself for experiencing the change and for taking the responsibility for making it happen.

These are some basic facts which I must again ask you to accept without question. Read these following statements over and over again several times:

- A relationship is not a static state. It is a constantly changing space in which there should be room to grow and experience new things constantly.
- For every doubt, concern and feeling of lack of fulfilment you are experiencing about your relationship, those people around you have as many doubts and are experiencing equal concern and lack of fulfilment.
- Unlike your conscious mind, your subconscious mind has no time reference. Whatever it was in the past that influences your behaviour patterns now could have happened a few moments ago as far as the subconscious mind is concerned. Therefore it is not necessary to go back into the past to deal with past painful experiences

or resurrect past pleasures. Pain can be dismissed instantly and pleasure revived instantly.

- In the Western world in particular, children are brought up to feel embarrassed and guilty about experiencing pleasures. Bearing in mind the previous statement, you can choose to dismiss this embarrassment and guilt immediately as if it had never existed.

- For every thought that you have ever had about improving or experimenting with your relationships, the people you know and are close to have had as many.

- Denying yourself pleasure is unkind and unnecessary, as is denying the same to other people in your life.

- Someone always has to make the first move. Take responsibility for this.

- Giving is power, not surrender.

- Whatever you give genuinely and unconditionally you will always get back severalfold.

### Exercise:

*I want you to carry out the following exercise today, please, and daily thereafter for three days.*

*Go to your favourite safe place in your home, lie back in a comfortable chair or on the bed or the floor and ensure that you will not be disturbed.*

### Stage One

*With the tip of your little finger and thumb pressed gently together, allow yourself to drift into the state that you would normally be after the first ten minutes of your PDP exercises. Release the pressure completely between your finger and thumb when you feel completely relaxed.*

### Stage Two

*Now I want you to identify one relationship in your life that you are unhappy with and picture this relationship as it is at its most uncomfortable or displeasing moments. Keep your eyes closed and create a picture of this in your mind. You may create this as a still picture or as a film. In either case, see it as brightly and as vividly in your mind as you can and as if it was actually happening at the time. If the picture or film is clearer and brighter in black and white, see it in black and white. If it is clearer and brighter in colour, then see it in colour. Make this picture as vivid as you possibly can.*

### Stage Three

*Now create another picture of this relationship precisely as you would like to see it and picture precisely what it is that*

you would need to do to improve it if you could drop all of
your inner defences, your embarrassment and your natural
tendency to hold back your feelings. Picture yourself doing
precisely that one thing. Once again this picture can be in
black and white or colour, still frame or in film form. Put
as much effort as you can into creating this scene.

### Stage Four

This is where you switch one picture for another in your
subconscious mind and this is how you do it.

First of all, make a large, vivid picture of the relationship
that you want to change or improve as you did in Stage
Two. Next, in the bottom right-hand corner of this
picture, make a small, dark version of the picture that you
created of how you can change this relationship.

Now switch the pictures. Take the small picture and in a
fraction of a second, blow it up in size. Make it bright and
vivid and see it in your mind bursting through your first
picture and exploding on to the screen in your mind. As
you do this and as the second picture bursts through the
screen, say out loud and in a powerful voice, 'WOW', and
hold that picture for at least five seconds.

Now open your eyes and close them again straight away
and repeat Stage Four again for a total of ten times. Open
your eyes for a second between each episode and do these
switches as quickly as you possibly can. Do not forget to
say 'WOW' each time that the new picture bursts through
the old.

*The very first time that you have the opportunity to recreate that scene in your life, take the opportunity and do so. Take the responsibility for making that happen. If the other person in that relationship does not react immediately as you would like or may have pictured, do not be concerned. You will have sown a strong seed in their subconscious mind and you will reap the benefits soon and as you wish them to be.*

## YOUR PSYCHO-DYNAMIC PROGRAMMING EXERCISES FOR THIS WEEK

### Morning PDP Exercises

First of all, carry out your twenty-minute relaxation and pre-programming exercise. At the end of this period, keeping your eyes closed, repeat the following statement silently to yourself and keep repeating it for a full ten minutes:

*'I (your name) will become my perfect weight and shape. I am positively happy with my life, my eating pattern and the way my relationships with everyone around me are improving. I feel good!'*

### Note:

*If you had to delay taking your Metabolic Test for a week due to your menstrual cycle and your temperature average was 97.4 degrees Fahrenheit or less, use the PDP Exercise One from last week in place of the above.*

### Evening PDP Exercises

Once again, go through the pre-programming exercise. At the end of this twenty-minute period, I want you to select another part of your body that you wish to improve the shape of. If this is a part of the body where you can tense and release the muscles without moving the rest of your body, then you should do so. If you can also reach those muscles comfortably and place your hands upon them and squeeze and release those muscles, do that. You must be able to do one or another of these whilst sitting or lying in a comfortable position.

*Now, and for the next ten minutes, I want you to picture yourself in a situation where you have enjoyed using those muscles before. Whatever time this was and whatever it was that you were doing, see this in your mind as clearly as you possibly can.*

## SUMMARY OF KEY POINTS

- Nothing affects the way you look more than the way you feel.
- You have the sole responsibility for how you feel – nobody can make you feel anything. You choose how you feel.
- There are three main food groups. These are fats, proteins and carbohydrates. Fats are a 'no-no'. Proteins are essential but the less dense they are in their natural state the better. Carbohydrates are the best source of energy, but test yourself for carbohydrate intolerance.
- If you have any of the health problems listed, turn to the appendix for the relevant support.
- Take careful note of and put into action the five Psycho-Slimming tips.
- Take full responsibility for improving your relationship with your partner. Use the PDP exercise to achieve this.
- Carry out your morning and evening PDP exercises.
- Complete your progress monitor chart at the end of this week.

## PROGRESS MONITOR – PLEASE COMPLETE AT THE END OF THE LAST DAY OF THE WEEK

**Instructions:**

Place a tick in the relevant column alongside each of the following questions. Do not think about your answers for too long – your initial reaction to each question will be the most accurate answer.

**Compared to when you first started this programme:**

| | worse | the same | better | much better | very much better | totally satisfied |
|---|---|---|---|---|---|---|
| How do you feel about your weight and shape now? | | | | | | |
| How do you think other people feel about your weight and shape now? | | | | | | |
| How do you feel about yourself as a person, taking into account factors such as your confidence, personality, sense of humour and ability to relate to and communicate with other people? | | | | | | |
| If you are in a close relationship with another person, how do you feel about this relationship now? | | | | | | |
| If you are in a close relationship with another person, how do you think that other person feels about this relationship now? | | | | | | |
| How do you feel about your confidence and ability to achieve your perfect weight and shape in the future and keep it there for ever? | | | | | | |
| How do you feel about being able to eat less, and more sensibly and nutritiously, in the future? | | | | | | |
| How do you feel about your ability to maintain any form of general exercise routine in the future? | | | | | | |

# CHAPTER FIVE

WEEK FIVE

# The Only Losers
# are the Quitters

## DEALING WITH SUCCESS

How were your progress monitor results last week? Almost certainly, there was an improvement noted against every weight-related and other 'feel-good' factor. If this programme is working for you, and I'm sure it is, then a few words of caution are necessary.

One of the most astounding things I discovered in my several years of private practice was just how many people actually enjoyed having problems and how they actually avoided success and the responsibility that it so often brings. If that seems surprising to you, think about it for a moment. It may well be that you are suffering from a similar condition and are not even aware of it.

Most people are brought up from early childhood to expect to experience a lifetime of problems. We are told by our parents that life is difficult and that we must learn to cope. We see our parents arguing over financial or career problems and when we question what is going on, are simply told that it is nothing for us to worry about now, we will have our own fair share later.

Have you ever heard the expression 'it's all a part of life's rich tapestry'? That expression is not referring to good, enriching experiences for us to enjoy; it relates only to bad ones for us to put up with and suffer.

How about when you were at school? Did you ever have cause to worry about what might happen to you if you did not get your homework in on time? Did you ever worry about not getting decent marks at the end of term exams and having your teacher haul you up in front of the class and make you feel small?

Do you ever worry about your job, your spouse, your children, your partner, what to have for dinner, what to buy when you go to the shops or how you are going to pay the bills?

Enough! I'm sure you could add another several hundred items to that list without any help from me at all. The plain fact of the matter is that most of us were brought up to believe that our lives would and should be difficult, that we were not put on this planet to have a good time and that we would always have something to worry about.

Is it any wonder that so many people shun success and have an underlying negative streak running right through their subconscious mind?

And the problems can get worse. Because of this childhood pre-programming, success and being positive can be very difficult for many people to cope with. Let's face it, when you have spent years learning to cope with worries and problems, they become almost second nature to you. You actually become quite comfortable with having them around you and you can fall back on them at any time and put the blame on them for your lack of success.

Success, on the other hand, can be very difficult to handle. Suddenly you have responsibilities. There is nobody you can put the blame on now. It is all down to you. This is not a comfortable feeling for many people.

Well, I am here to tell you that to expect a life of stress and worry is absolute nonsense. You were put on this earth to be successful, to be free of worries, to enjoy life to its fullest extent and to help others do the same. You are here to earn as much money as you want if that is what you want, to have a really good time and to enjoy everything that nature put on this earth for you.

There is another reason for me to be congratulating you now, no matter how large or small the level of improvement you have made, and this is this week's big surprise. Are you ready?

## YOU ARE ALREADY YOUR PERFECT WEIGHT AND SIZE – CONGRATULATIONS. YOU'VE WON!!!!

Before you assume I am joking with you, let me assure you that I am not. For the moment and for as long as you choose this moment to last, you are your perfect weight and shape. This minute that you are living in and experiencing right now is the only one you will ever have in your whole life. You have had other minutes before and will have many other minutes in the future, but you will only ever have this one minute.

## LIVING IN REAL TIME

Most people spend most of their lives either living in the past or living in the future. They are so preoccupied with what they did yesterday, the day before that and the year before that, and so busy planning or worrying about the future, that they never get time to appreciate the minute that they are living in. How much time do you spend living in the 'right now this minute'?

Think about it for a moment. How much time did you spend yesterday living in the past? Did you waste any of your 'now' minutes recalling a conversation that you had with somebody that either upset you or concerned you in case you might have upset them? How many times in the past have you wasted precious time going back over past conversations in your head and wishing you had said something else to score a point or make your point more clearly? Why did you waste your time? The other person had forgotten the conversation long before you dragged it up in your mind again.

How many people spent an hour yesterday lying on the psychiatrist's couch having their long-gone past dragged up in order to try and help them deal with situations in the future, and, in the process, wasted another precious couple of hours? And how much time did they waste beforehand worrying about what would happen at the session? And yes, I do mean wasted. There is no need to spend weeks or months delving into the past and reliving your childhood problems in order to change the future when as much, if not more, can be achieved in a few minutes using Psycho-Dynamic Programming techniques.

How much time do you personally spend thinking about things that happened in the past that are unpleasant rather than pleasant to recall and so miss all those precious things that are happening around you while you are somewhere in the distant past?

The past is the past and the future is the future, and yet for every hour that you have spent living in the past, you probably have spent at least ten times that amount of time worrying about the future. Will you pass those exams? Has your boyfriend given you up because it is now ten minutes past eight and he said he would call at eight? How many precious minutes did you waste fretting and worrying until he eventually called? Have you ever sat for hours worrying why your partner was late home from work or the children late home from school when you could have been spending those precious moments walking around your garden and appreciating the trees and the flowers and those other precious gifts of nature?

Have you ever sat up at night worrying if you or your partner would get the promotion you were after, or how you were going to pay the bills, or a thousand other things? What a waste of time! How many times did your worst fears ever become a reality and did the worrying do anything to help?

How much time have you spent worrying about your weight and shape in the past and how much have you wasted in the last few weeks worrying about what it will be in the future? Have you been to the gymnasium today – or been doing any exercises – and been thinking about the past or the future instead of enjoying the experience of your body and your surroundings?

No, I am not in any way deriding this programme. But let me also make it quite clear that if I did not know that you were going to get a lot more out of this book than just achieving your perfect weight and shape, I would not have written it in the first place.

Let us assume that this minute you are in now is the only minute that you will ever have in your whole life. Would you choose to spend it being concerned about your weight and shape? Would you worry about the cellulite at the top of your thighs or the fact that your bottom was a little too large and your neck was too thick? Of course you would not. You would make sure that you got some pleasure out of this minute!

And if you were lucky and got an extra minute, you would do the same, would you not?

Well, that is just how life is. One minute after another, until something or somebody says that you have had enough minutes and it is all over. So is your weight really worth worrying about? Can you accept that for just this minute you are your perfect weight and shape? Choose to do that, please.

Of course there is nothing wrong with planning for the future, as long as you are not living in it. Planning is good common sense and can be a very useful and enjoyable part of your life. And planning to achieve a different perfect weight and shape in the future from the one you have this minute and enjoying the process and enjoying the way you are now at the same time is wonderful.

Why did I not tell you four weeks ago that you were already your perfect weight and shape? You have every right to ask. But four weeks ago you would have found it far more difficult to accept. It is only because of your PDP exercises and the other techniques that you have learned that your mind is now able to accept this statement instead of rejecting it. So are you not pleased that I held back for a little while? Think of all the other valuable things that you have learned and are going to learn.

So you are already your perfect weight and shape for this minute. You have scored an increase again across most if not all of the 'feel-good' factors, and many of you may already have decided that you are now as you wish to be in the future. If you wish, and as a result of what we have just discussed, you can go back and alter last week's progress monitor chart.

You are also a lot more positive about many other aspects of your life and maybe you are thinking that you have done enough and can quit this programme. If that is so, remember my opening statement at the beginning of this week.

'The only losers are the quitters!'

You are well over halfway through this programme, and by the time you have finished it, I know you will want to carry on using many of the techniques you have learned throughout the rest of your life. So no quitting. If you so choose, your weight and shape can be far more perfect than they currently are and you can learn to get even more enjoyment out of life.

*Exercise:*
This week I want you to take part in a very special exercise. You are going to find it a strange and wonderful experience and one that will change the way you think about your life and live your life for ever. This week you are going to focus entirely on living in the now.

First of all, retrieve the second set of twenty-five coloured labels you bought two weeks ago and write the word 'NOW' on every one. Once again, place these in different places where your conscious mind and your subconscious mind will see them frequently throughout the day, but do not put them in the same places as your previous labels. Save one of these labels for this first exercise.

Now place the remaining label on a sheet of stiff white paper, seat yourself in a comfortable chair and balance the sheet of paper on your lap so that it is clearly visible to you and you can see it without straining.

Close your eyes and go through your pre-programming exercise for just ten minutes. Then open your eyes and stare intently at the label on your piece of paper and repeat the following statement over and over again for a full ten minutes:

'I (your name) am living in the now. The past and the future are irrelevant now. This minute and every minute is mine to appreciate and enjoy now. I am already my perfect weight and shape.'

*During this exercise, it is inevitable that your eyes will become out of focus because of your concentration on the label. That is fine. Do not attempt to bring the label back into focus. Whatever happens in this ten minutes is meant to be happening.*

You will be using this same exercise for your morning PDP exercise for the rest of this week. If you find it as enjoyable as many people do, you may repeat this as frequently as you wish throughout the day, and if you choose to do that, you need only carry out five minutes of the pre-programming exercise on these occasions.

For the rest of this week, I want you to concentrate entirely on living in the now and enjoying every minute of the week, minute by minute. Enjoy your food and savour every mouthful. Enjoy your exercise in whatever form you take it. Enjoy and savour everything that is going on around you as if it were a wonderful gift that you may never see again. Do not waste any opportunity to enjoy what you are doing. Any time you find yourself drifting back into the past or worrying about the future instead of planning to enjoy the future, remind yourself that for this week at least, you are going to focus on living in the 'now'.

## FURTHER IMPROVING YOUR RELATIONSHIPS
Enjoying better and more fulfilling relationships is one of life's great healers. There is great scope for improving your relationships and therefore everything in your life if you take the responsibility for this.

Once again, some more facts that you will have to take my word for. We have no time for detailed explanations, but I can assure you that the following 'Nine Golden Guides' that I am about to give you are based on several years of working with people just like you. These people are now enjoying more fulfilling relationships, thanks to the Golden Guides. They apply equally to all the people close to you in your life as well as the closest of those relationships. So why go through what can be a painful experience yourself when you can learn from other people's experiences?

## THE NINE GOLDEN GUIDES

### Golden Guide One

A relationship is not a fixed menu from which you select the items of behaviour that you want at any given time. It is a constantly changing environment in which to experiment and grow. This applies equally to both people in the relationship.

Choose to accept the limitless boundaries that should be a natural feature of your relationships.

### Golden Guide Two

Whenever you are experiencing dissatisfaction with your relationship, consciously or subconsciously, the other person is feeling equally dissatisfied. You do not need to voice your problem for that person to know that something is wrong. Your feelings are broadcast almost like a radio signal. Their subconscious mind will pick up your feelings automatically. Because they do not consciously know that it is your dissatisfaction that they are feeling, they believe they are feeling dissatisfied about something in the relationship themselves.

You experience the same feelings when they are transmitting their conscious or subconscious thoughts.

Choose to discuss your feelings openly. Do not blame your feelings on them. Own your feelings and express them. By so doing you will be sending out a clear message which they can help you with instead of them receiving a subconscious and unclear message.

## Golden Guide Three

The people that you surround yourself with are precisely the people that you need to be with at this moment in your life in order to make it whole. They are your partners in life. The same applies to them: they need you just as much as you need them.

## Golden Guide Four

When you first start out in a relationship, both partners act out a courtship ritual. This applies to most types of relationships and especially so to romantic ones. You choose to do a lot of things that you would not normally do to establish and enhance the relationship, and you often particularly enjoy the relationship at this stage. It is not, however, a state that you or that other person are intending or are able to maintain. Yet you can retrieve this state for periods of time if you choose to take responsibility for bringing it into the 'now' instead of keeping it in the past. The more frequently you do this, the longer those periods will last.

**Golden Guide Five**
We spend so much time during our childhood and throughout our lifetimes being denied the comforts we need to create our own feelings of security that denial becomes our major tool to express our dissatisfactions. It is our partners in our relationships that are denied what they need by us and they in turn use that same tool against us.

You have needs that must be fulfilled for you to be happy and fulfilled. So do your partners. Choose to provide these needs for them. If your relationships are such that you have forgotten or never knew what your partners' real needs are, then ask.

Giving your partners what you know they need will give you pleasure and you will receive as much if not more in return. Your needs will also be fulfilled.

**Golden Guide Six**
Life is full of surprises. Unfortunately many of them can be unpleasant. If you would like to experience only pleasant surprises, choose to let go and behave as you want, when you want, without inhibition. You will get a delightful surprise when you experience how good this can feel and your partners will be subconsciously driven to do the same.

**Golden Guide Seven**
There are some things that your partners enjoy doing that you have never been able to enjoy in the past and some that you would not join in with. The same goes for your partners.

Choose to give in and allow yourself to join in and appreciate them. By so doing, you will find that your partners will reciprocate.

**Golden Guide Eight**
Your partners are your friends and allies, not your enemies. Choose to treat them as such.

**Golden Guide Nine**
Somebody always has to start the ball rolling in order to achieve anything. Your partners may not have had the benefit of participating in this programme or benefiting from the techniques of Psycho-Dynamic Programming. You have, and it is therefore you who must take the responsibility for changing your relationships. You will experience a great joy by doing so.

Please read these Nine Golden Guides every day this week at least twice a day.

## WATER CAN BE YOUR BEST FRIEND
Water is the staff of life. Without food, your body can survive for many days and even weeks. Without water you die very quickly.

Water bathes the cells throughout all your internal organs and tissues. It washes them clean of waste materials and poisons and refreshes them, just as it does the outside of your body when you take a shower.

Water also helps in the proper digestion of your food, can act as a regular 'pick-me-up' throughout the day and makes your brain more alert and positive. And of course a glass of water half an hour before a meal can help to reduce your appetite.

Water is also a natural medicine and has been used for centuries in various forms for the treatment of a wide range of illnesses and debilitating conditions. One of the most invaluable aspects of water as a medicine is the fact that it works in conjunction with your body's natural healing systems. Unlike drugs and other medicines, many of which actually damage good cells whilst trying to seek out and destroy the bad cells, water always has a positive effect and enhances the body's natural inclination to heal itself.

**Water Therapy**
There are two things that I would like you to do with water from now on. The first is not optional; it must be done. The second is optional, but after the first time you experience it, I am sure that you will want to do it every day.

The first is to drink more water. Drink a glass first thing every morning and another glass about half an hour before every meal. In addition to that, substitute a glass of water for another beverage that you may be consuming frequently throughout the day. That does not mean that you should give up drinking tea or coffee. The caffeine content in these drinks can act as a weight loss aid. Nevertheless, replace some of these or other drinks you might take with a glass of cool, clear water and make sure that you drink at least six glasses a day.

## Cold Water Walking

Have you ever taken a walk along the side of the beach with your feet immersed up to your ankles in the sea? If you have then you know that the effects can be euphoric. It is the water that is creating this feeling. The surroundings that you are in may heighten the experience, but it is the water and the action of your feet within it that create the feelings you experience. This is the second part of your water therapy.

*Exercise:*
*Here is what you do. Fill your bath with cold water to ankle depth. If you do not have a bath, block the water run-away in your shower and let the shower basin fill to the same depth. Then steady yourself with one hand against a convenient support and walk on the spot for three to five minutes as if you were walking along a beach. When you have finished this exercise, dry your feet vigorously with a towel.*

*You will find this exercise refreshing and extremely energising. In addition to these effects, it will also help to improve your resistance to disease and will stimulate your circulation, which in itself will help you to achieve an even more perfect weight and shape.*

## Watery Foods

It is not by accident that some of the foods that are best for the body have a high water content. Foods that contain a lot of water are extremely good for you, so choose to eat plenty of vegetables, fruits and other 'wet' foods.

## *YOUR PSYCHO-DYNAMIC PROGRAMMING EXERCISES FOR THIS WEEK*

### *Morning PDP Exercises*

*Carry out your twenty-minute pre-programming exercise. After this exercise, repeat the following statement, which was mentioned earlier in this chapter. Do this for a full ten minutes.*

*'I (your name) am living in the now. The past and the future are irrelevant now. This minute and every minute is mine to appreciate and enjoy now. I am already my perfect weight and shape.'*

### *Evening PDP Exercises*

*Once again, carry out your pre-programming exercises. When you have done this, repeat the following statement over and over again for a full ten minutes.*

*'I (your name) am already my perfect weight and shape and this can be more perfect in the future if I choose. I take the responsibility for making the relationship with my partner more perfect also.'*

*If you are not currently in a relationship with a partner, substitute the following statement:*

*'I (your name) am already my perfect weight and shape and this can be more perfect in the future if I choose. I take the responsibility for making my relationships with all other people more perfect also.'*

## SUMMARY OF KEY POINTS

- You were put upon this earth to enjoy it. Do so.
- You are already your perfect weight and shape for now and this can be more perfect in the future if you choose.
- No matter how satisfied you are with your weight and shape, continue with this programme.
- Practise 'living in the now'.
- Read your 'Nine Golden Guides' every day this week, at least twice a day. Read them slowly and understand and think about what you are reading.
- Drink at least six glasses of cool, clear water every day. One of these should be taken approximately half an hour before meals.
- Do your cold water walking exercise every morning and in the evenings also, if you wish.
- Carry out your morning and evening PDP exercises and the additional PDP exercise every day.
- Complete your progress monitor chart at the end of this week.

**PROGRESS MONITOR – PLEASE COMPLETE AT THE END OF THE LAST DAY OF THE WEEK**

Instructions:

Place a tick in the relevant column alongside each of the following questions. Do not think about your answers for too long – your initial reaction to each question will be the most accurate answer.

Compared to when you first started this programme:

| | worse | the same | better | much better | very much better | totally satisfied |
|---|---|---|---|---|---|---|
| How do you feel about your weight and shape now? | | | | | | |
| How do you think other people feel about your weight and shape now? | | | | | | |
| How do you feel about yourself as a person, taking into account factors such as your confidence, personality, sense of humour and ability to relate to and communicate with other people? | | | | | | |
| If you are in a close relationship with another person, how do you feel about this relationship now? | | | | | | |
| If you are in a close relationship with another person, how do you think that other person feels about this relationship now? | | | | | | |
| How do you feel about your confidence and ability to achieve your perfect weight and shape in the future and keep it there for ever? | | | | | | |
| How do you feel about being able to eat less, and more sensibly and nutritiously, in the future? | | | | | | |
| How do you feel about your ability to maintain any form of general exercise routine in the future? | | | | | | |

# CHAPTER SIX

## WEEK SIX

# Melt Down

Although this may be the last chapter of this book, this is not the last week in your programme.

The last five weeks have been your introduction into a new programme or phase in your life. You can continue with this programme for as long as you wish. At the end of this week I will show you how to use the information you have learned and your Psycho-Dynamic Programming exercises in order for you to continue to make progress in any field of activity that you choose.

## FIRE WATER

We finished up our programme last week discussing water and how useful it can be in helping you to achieve your perfect weight and shape. There is another type of water we need to talk about, and this one is in a form that can hinder you from achieving your final 'melt down'. It used to be called 'fire water'. You would know it as alcohol, and if there is one thing that every weight-control or weight-reducing programme agrees upon, it is that excess alcohol is not on the menu.

Because I think that this subject is so important, not only in terms of achieving your future perfect weight or anything else you have decided to be successful with, I am going to give you more background information on this than I have done on many other subjects that we have covered over the last few weeks.

Background information aside, if you want to have a more perfect weight and shape in the future than you have now, then alcohol is another 'no-no' or, at least, a 'no-no, one is enough, thank you'. If you believe that you are carbohydrate intolerant, then alcohol should definitely not be on the menu at all.

Alcohol is, quite simply, raw calories. There is no other type of food that the body absorbs so quickly and turns into fat so rapidly. Alcohol makes fat!

I appreciate that we live in a society where alcohol is considered so much the norm that it is almost more difficult to say 'no' to another drink than to another helping of dessert. I also appreciate that the conviviality of enjoying a drink with a few friends can be one of life's most relaxing and entertaining experiences. However, before you make up your mind about how much or how little you are going to drink in the future, let me tell you about Peter.

## Peter's Story
Peter came to consult me because, for some months, he had been feeling particularly tired, and anything other than going through the motions of doing his job reasonably well was just too much of an effort.

Peter's doctor had dismissed the problem as being tiredness due to overwork, but Peter knew this was not the case. If anything, the complete opposite was the truth.

Peter was actually working a lot less than he had ever done before and he did not have the strength to do anything else. And his subconscious mind knew that there was something wrong. At forty-five years of age, he was beginning to feel very old.

Peter's day went something like this. He would get up at about six-thirty in the morning. He would normally skip breakfast in favour of two cups of coffee to get himself going and rush to leave home in order to miss the early morning traffic. When he arrived at his desk, it was usually piled high with the remains of several unfinished projects. He would have another two or three cups of coffee to try and raise his energy levels and make a start on clearing the backlog of work. During the course of the morning, he would have another few cups of coffee.

He invariably skipped lunch altogether or, at most, grabbed a hurried sandwich. If he was lunching with a client, this was always a disaster. Most of his clients drank alcohol before and during their meal and Peter would drink to be sociable. When he did, he felt so ineffectual a few hours later that there was little point in him going back to the office, although he almost always did.

Because he was feeling so tired, Peter had given up his normal, after-office work-out at the gymnasium and had replaced this with a stop en route for home at the local pub. Two or three beers later, he felt uplifted and better for a while. When he got home he would have a good evening meal and usually accompany this with half a bottle of wine, or possibly more, before crashing out in front of the television. He was often in bed by nine or nine-thirty.

And the following day he would start this routine all over again. Does this pattern seem familiar to you?

Peter did not think his drinking was excessive. He knew many people who drank an awful lot more than he did and he certainly did not think of himself as an alcoholic. But, as Peter put it, 'Drinking does give me a lift much quicker and more easily than anything else I can do, and I do admit that my drinking has been getting slowly and progressively heavier'.

I sent Peter to another doctor to have a series of blood tests done and the results were as I had suspected. There were slight liver function abnormalities, but other than that, he was fine. Or was he?

Peter had always prided himself on his youthful looks and had appeared to be at least eight years younger than his actual age. He had all his hair and was reasonably good-looking. He had a lot of pride, too, and was concerned that he was starting to look older and feel older. He also did not like the fact that he had put a lot of weight on around his middle and had been forced into buying new shirts because his neck had thickened out. Fortunately for Peter, he was not prepared to give in to ageing so quickly.

Peter's situation was actually a lot worse than he first thought. He exhibited many of the symptoms of carbohydrate intolerance, he was drinking far too much for his body weight and, as far as I was concerned, was drinking himself into early old age and probably premature death.

We used the same PDP exercise that you will find in the appendix and Peter stopped drinking instantly. In just a few months, Peter lost weight, regained most of his youthful looks, felt a lot better and was really back on top of his job. In fact, he gained an unexpected promotion and he ran in the New York marathon that year.

Why is Peter's story so important to you? There are two reasons. In the first place, it illustrates the potential danger of excess alcohol in terms of weight gain, loss of energy and ambition and the ultimate danger of alcoholism and even premature death. Equally as important is how Peter felt about giving up alcohol.

Like most people, Peter associated alcohol with social pleasures and social occasions. Before his PDP exercises, he could not perceive himself saying 'no' to a pint of lager or a large gin and tonic in favour of a glass of fizzy water. But now Peter takes great pride in doing so. He gets a great kick out of telling people that he does not drink and enjoys their questions as to why not. He also likes the looks of puzzlement and admiration that he always gets. Peter knows that many of his friends and colleagues envy his abstinence and wish they could also be different. .

Peter used to feel more sociable, less inhibited and much better company when he had drunk a few large gin and tonics. He feels even better now and gets as much of a kick out of not drinking as he did when he was drinking. He is just as sociable and a lot more fun. It is a different sort of kick and, to Peter, it is a much better one.

I have no problem with you having some alcohol whilst on this programme, particularly as by now, you realise that this is a programme for life. I do not even mind if you go out on a really wild binge from time to time. However, you do need to remember that excess alcohol makes you fat. Excess alcohol can also cause premature ageing of all the body cells, including your brain cells and your skin cells. You think older, look older and get older, faster. Excess alcohol, particularly taken on a regular basis, can lead to alcoholism and can contribute to heart disease, liver disease, some forms of cancer, senility, anxiety and depression and a host of other problems.

And as for keeping to any type of programme, whether it be work, something in your social calendar or your programme to achieve more out of life and attain your future perfect weight and shape, it is a lot more difficult keeping to anything when you have a hangover!

You too can make the same choice as Peter and you have the tools to achieve this if you wish. Go to the relevant exercise if you need help.

## COMFORT EATING
Comfort eating is not an uncommon problem. Many people choose to eat or drink when they feel uncomfortable or bored with something that is going on in their lives. It is often so much easier to get comfort from some favourite food or drink than it is to face up to the problem and do something about it. The comfort is always short-lived and, inevitably, the same feelings come rushing back afterwards, often at two to three times higher than their previous level.

Again, you now have all the tools to deal with comfort eating. You are already more positive, more successful and more able to deal with any situation that you choose to deal with. All you have to do is to make that choice, or allow your subconscious mind to make the choice by utilising your PDP exercises. The person you now feel most comfortable with to help you deal with any uncomfortable feelings you may have is you.

## YOUR BODY'S INTERNAL FAT FURNACE

You have a secret weapon in your body that can help you to achieve a more perfect weight and shape in the future. This secret weapon consists of a group of highly specialised cells called 'brown fat cells', which are located predominantly down the sides of the bones which make up your neck and spine.

Brown fat cells are totally different to the fat cells you have in your body which account for your excess weight and the bulges in the various places that you do not want them. The type of fat that is found in these places is a yellow fat and is the result of your overeating, eating the wrong foods and lack of exercise.

Each brown fat cell is like a little mini-furnace. It is packed full of a number of chemicals whose responsibility it is to take in excess calories, burn them up and dissipate them as heat. If you have ever experienced going to bed soon after a heavy meal and a few drinks and waking up a few hours later feeling terribly hot, you now know that is the result of your brown fat cells going to work on your food to try and get rid of the calories that your body is unable to use in any other way.

There are various ways that you can speed up the brown fat cell activity in your body and help it to burn up those extra calories.

In the first place, there are several foods that contain ingredients that can speed up the metabolism and activity of your brown cells. These ingredients are the amino acid called Tyrosine and the minerals Iodine, Copper and Zinc. The section in the appendix dealing with nutritional support will give you the best food sources of these nutrients.

Caffeine can also have a stimulating effect on brown fat cell activity, but there is no need to consume large quantities. In fact, over a certain level of caffeine intake, say three to four cups of medium-strength black coffee a day, there can be an opposite effect. So three to four cups of coffee a day should be the maximum.

There are also certain foods that can have an adverse effect on the activity of your brown cells and these are the denser and less digestible forms of protein that we discussed in an earlier chapter. I'm sorry to have to mention it again, but it is another good reason for cutting down on your consumption of meat. These less digestible proteins can work their way into the brown fat cells and effectively poison them. The more dense protein you eat, the longer lasting is the effect of this poisoning.

Aerobic exercise can also have a dramatic effect on speeding up the rate at which your brown fat cells can burn up calories, and I presume that, by now, you have established a fifteen- to twenty-minute aerobic exercise routine that you are doing most days.

Knowing how I work by now, you may also have guessed that there is another form of exercise that you can use to increase your brown fat cell activity, and of course you are right. We have a PDP exercise to help you achieve this, and I would like you to try this out every morning this week as part of your normal programme.

*Exercise:*
*Sit in a comfortable chair and carry out your five-minute deep breathing exercise and five minutes of your relaxation exercise whilst keeping the tip of your little finger and thumb pressed gently together.*

*When you have completed this ten minutes, release your finger and thumb.*

*I now want you to picture all those masses of brown fat cells along the sides of your neck bones and spine. See them as golden brown in colour and glowing. When you have a clear picture of this in your mind, I want you to see them suddenly become alive. I want you to picture the brown cells at the top of your neck, golden and glowing, suddenly start throbbing and pulsing with activity and burning with white-hot intensity. I want you to see this activity of the brown cells spreading slowly down your neck and right to the base of your spine until the whole area is a throbbing, pulsating, glowing mass of golden, hot energy.*

*As you visualise this reaching the base of your spine you will feel a tingling sensation and as soon as you experience this, press the tip of your finger and thumb together again.*

This part of the exercise should take no more than ten minutes and is the most effective way of increasing the ability of your brown fat cells to help you to achieve your perfect weight and shape in the future.

## HOW IS YOUR OTHER PROGRAMME GOING?

A few weeks ago I asked you to take your first step to doing something else in your life that was important to you. How is it going? Did you even take that first step? If you did, then remember that 'the only losers are the quitters'. You should be taking your second, third and fourth steps by now.

If you have not even taken your first, then it is not too late to do so. Here are some examples to encourage you.

One of my wealthy ex-clients who used to have a gardener in to do her gardening decided to get involved in a little of the activity herself. She gave up sitting on the patio in her best frock, entertaining her friends with a glass of wine, and exchanged the frock for a pair of dungarees and some gardening gloves. She started small with a few packets of seeds and some seed trays. She is now heavily involved with the local branch of her gardening society and speaks regularly and demonstrates flower arranging at venues all over the country. It took one small step to start.

Joe was an overweight office junior in the City. He worked in a busy dealing room and was about to quit, since the pressure put upon him by his high-powered peers was just too much for him to cope with. Joe used PDP techniques and made the decision to choose to stand up for himself and be counted as a valuable member of the team. Two years later he has not lost a great deal of his excess weight, but he does not feel it is important to do so and is very happy with his weight the way it is. He is also leading the team now. He runs the department!

Mary claimed to be too busy to do anything. Most of her spare time was spent running the children backwards and forwards to school and taking them to various other locations for their extra-curricular activities. Mary took her first step by organising a mini-cab to take and deliver her children and three of her children's friends to school. The additional cost was little compared to the extra free time that she gained. Mary also learned a lot more from that exercise. Instead of being the 'not very bright' housewife that she thought she was, she found that she had excellent organisational abilities. She also learned that other people listened to her and respected her opinions, something that she had never dreamed of in the past.

Four years later, Mary now runs her own business. She leases four small coaches, employs six part-time drivers and has contracts with two local schools. As well as running her business, she is also a valued member of the local Chamber of Commerce and is involved with several local charities. Everything that Mary has achieved started with one small step.

So whether you are taking your first step or the next of many, do it, keep to it and let your subconscious mind take you forward. Nothing is impossible. Don't let any-one else's conscious mind or your own ever tell you that you cannot do something. You can do anything that you choose to do. If you doubt this in any way, let me assure you that you do have the power.

## POWER WHENEVER YOU NEED IT

The following exercise has been taught to thousands of people and I know of none for whom it has not worked. It will enable you to harness all your hidden and potential power whenever and wherever you need it and allow you to step beyond the boundaries of any previous limitations you may have thought that you had.

*Exercise:*
Go to a place where you can be alone. Stand upright and erect with your chin up, your shoulders back, and with your back straight. Take a few seconds to absorb how good this feels.

Now I want you to go back to a time when you felt at your most powerful. Close your eyes and picture that scene. It may have been many years ago when you were at school and taking part in the school sports day. You may have been first over the winning line and you can hear the crowds cheering, feel the tears of joy running down your face and feel yourself bursting with pride, joy and exhilaration.

It may have been at the birth stage of your pregnancy. If you felt more powerful and wonderful then than at any other time in your life, picture that now.

It could have been the day you came back from an interview and had got your first job. It may be the time you received that first and most important promotion.

Whatever that most powerful occasion was, imagine it now in every detail and with all of your senses. Feel the excitement and the tingling sensation throughout your body.

Next, hold out your strong hand in front of you, palm facing upwards, and imagine those feelings pouring into the palm of your hand. Hear the sounds that were going on around you at the time and pour those sounds into your palm as well. See everything that was happening and pour the memories into your outstretched hand.

138

*When you are feeling this experience at its most illuminating and exciting moment, clench your fist and capture the feelings in your hand. At the same time as you clench your fist, say in a loud and powerful voice the word 'YES'. Say it with power.*

In the future, whenever you need extra power to help you achieve anything – whether it is the next step in your other programme, or when you need the strength to say no to a second helping of dessert or another or even your first drink – clench your fist and, if appropriate, say 'yes' out loud and with that same power. If the circumstances are such that other people might think this strange and you might feel it embarrassing, then say it within yourself quietly and with power. It will have an equal effect.

You can also increase the power at your disposal. Whenever you achieve something else that makes you feel good and powerful, take the opportunity to pour those new feelings into that same palm and clench your fist over them. Say 'yes' again and trap that extra power for future use.

## WHAT ELSE DO YOU NEED TO KNOW?
I shall start by answering that question in the way that you probably expected me to by now. Your subconscious mind already knew all the answers that you needed to know in order for you to achieve your perfect weight and shape. All that you really needed to know was how to tap into the subconscious mind and use that knowledge to enable you to make things happen for you.

The real function of any psychologist or psychiatrist should be to help you to realise things for yourself, not to tell them to you. Unfortunately for most people, they do not have the knowledge of the techniques of Psycho-Dynamic Programming to enable them to achieve this as fast as they might wish. Indeed, many people spend years on the psychiatrist's couch, often getting a lot worse before they ever get any better. This need not happen to you. Your subconscious mind already knew everything that it needed to know in order for you to achieve anything that you wanted in your life. Your subconscious is now very much sharper and more active on your behalf than it was before. Your conscious mind also has a lot of new information to assist you.

You have also learned several other facts that will help you to achieve your perfect weight and shape in the future if you wish to improve on what you have achieved so far.

What else do you need to know? Only that you have my continued support now and for ever in the future. In the following section I will show you how to design your own PDP programmes, and this book and the techniques that it contains can be your guide and companion for the future.

## *YOUR PSYCHO-DYNAMIC PROGRAMMING EXERCISES FOR THIS WEEK*

### *Morning PDP Exercise*
*Your morning PDP exercise has already been explained to you a few pages back.*

### *Evening PDP Exercises*
*Carry out the pre-programming exercises and relaxation exercises as you have been doing for the last five weeks. This is the last week that you will need to spend twenty minutes doing this.*

*When you have completed this twenty-minute stage, repeat the following statement over and over again for a full ten minutes:*

*'I (your name) am the power to achieve anything and everything that I want in my life.'*

## SUMMARY OF KEY POINTS

- Reduce your consumption of alcohol to a minimum. If you believe that you have an intolerance to carbohydrates, give it up altogether. You will be surprised and delighted at how much better you feel.
- Brown fat cells burn up excess calories. Use the nutritional guidance notes contained in the appendix, physical exercise and your PDP exercises to activate your brown fat cells.
- Make sure that you take steps to start and continue with your other programme of achievement. Take one small step at a time.
- Use the clenched fist technique to harness and increase your personal power.
- Your subconscious mind already knew everything that you needed to know in order for you to achieve your perfect weight and shape and anything else that you wanted to achieve. Your conscious mind now knows this also.
- Carry out your morning and evening PDP exercises.
- Complete your progress monitor chart at the end of this week.

**PROGRESS MONITOR – PLEASE COMPLETE AT THE END OF THE LAST DAY OF THE WEEK**

Instructions:

Place a tick in the relevant column alongside each of the following questions. Do not think about your answers for too long – your initial reaction to each question will be the most accurate answer.

Compared to when you first started this programme:

| | worse | the same | better | much better | very much better | totally satisfied |
|---|---|---|---|---|---|---|
| How do you feel about your weight and shape now? | | | | | | |
| How do you think other people feel about your weight and shape now? | | | | | | |
| How do you feel about yourself as a person, taking into account factors such as your confidence, personality, sense of humour and ability to relate to and communicate with other people? | | | | | | |
| If you are in a close relationship with another person, how do you feel about this relationship now? | | | | | | |
| If you are in a close relationship with another person, how do you think that other person feels about this relationship now? | | | | | | |
| How do you feel about your confidence and ability to achieve your perfect weight and shape in the future and keep it there for ever? | | | | | | |
| How do you feel about being able to eat less, and more sensibly and nutritiously, in the future? | | | | | | |
| How do you feel about your ability to maintain any form of general exercise routine in the future? | | | | | | |

# Summary

**WHICH CATEGORY ARE YOU?**
By the time you have reached this section of the book you will have fallen into one of two categories.

If you are in the first category, you will have already achieved your perfect weight and shape and will also have made your own decision as to how you want to be and what else you want to achieve in the future. For that, I am proud of you and I thank you for your cooperation. Unless we have people completing this programme successfully, then other people will be less likely to embark upon it in the future.

If you come into the second category, then you have probably read through this book quickly from start to finish. It certainly will not have taken you six weeks.

You know, or your subconscious mind is telling you, that although some of the techniques that you have read about seem rather strange, they will work. You will have tested a few but not quite wholeheartedly. In spite of that, you have still experienced some unusual thoughts and sensations. You also know that everything else that you have read makes more sense than probably anything else that you have learned about losing weight before.

You will also be more than a little interested in achieving some other aims and ambitions in your life. So what are you going to do now? Are you going to put this book to one side until you have a 'spare' six weeks? Let me

144

assure you that you never will have. Either start right now or give up the idea altogether.

## I DARE YOU!

Do you remember when you were a child at school and somebody dared you to do something? I am sure that it happened to you and that you responded to the dare for one of two reasons. Either there was a reward in it for you because the person doing the daring was hoping that you might hurt yourself and get into trouble, or the darer would have claimed that you were a coward and you did not want to lose face.

I don't suppose you fall for dares any more, do you?

## WELL, I DARE YOU!

If you fall into the second category I described, I dare you to go back to page one and start this programme all over again right now. The difference is that I do not want you to get into trouble, and being overweight can be trouble.

I also do not want you to lose face. This programme works, and every other one you have tried has not. It is almost certain that you have told people about this book, in spite of my request for you not to. I do not want you to have to look at any person ever again, including yourself in the mirror, and have to say to yourself or anyone else that you failed. You can choose to be a winner right now by starting again. What do you have to lose other than your dissatisfaction with your current weight and shape?

If you have kept to this programme or accept my dare to go back and start again, we want to know of your success. Please do drop a note to me, care of the publisher, whose address can be found at the front of this book. A copy of the last week of your progress monitor chart would also be helpful. Thank you!

### Living Your Life – Not Living a Life

You are here for around three score years and ten. That is approximately thirty-seven million 'now' minutes.

If, as we discussed earlier, you choose to live and enjoy every one of those thirty-seven million minutes, you are going to have a wonderful life and those people that you share it with will benefit from just being with you.

Think about that for a moment. Thirty-seven million minutes of beauty, love, enjoyment, excitement and appreciation of life to the full. Is this what you have chosen for yourself? If not, it is not too late to make that choice.

### HOW TO USE PSYCHO-DYNAMIC PROGRAMMING IN THE FUTURE

The techniques of PDP are not difficult to follow and put into practice every day of your life, and they can be used to achieve all manner of things.

I mentioned earlier that by the time you had come to the end of week six you would no longer need to carry out the pre-programming exercises for the full twenty minutes in the future, and this is now the case. However, it will help to keep your subconscious mind on the alert if you do the exercises at least twice a week. For the rest of the time, you can use the following exercise to put your mind almost immediately into the state that it needs to be to put your new messages into your subconscious mind.

*Exercise:*
*The following exercise is to be used in the future prior to any 'I' statements that you choose to make.*

*Find a quiet, comfortable place and carry out the five minutes of your breathing exercise. In the last minute only, touch the tip of your little finger and thumb together and squeeze these gently for the remaining minute of the exercise. That is now all you need to do.*

*If you are still seeking to achieve a more perfect weight and shape, or just need reassurance and reminding of what you have learned to do in order to achieve this, use any of the statements that are most appropriate and that you felt most comfortable with when you used them before. Whichever you select, use that one and only that one for at least three days and use it morning and evening. Do not be tempted to change it or try and use more than one at a time in the future. There is no hurry any more.*

## ACHIEVING OTHER THINGS

What about the other things that you want to achieve and be successful at? You can use PDP exercises to achieve almost anything that you want, whether it is something material that you wish to own; something that it is realistic for you to want to achieve given a reasonable time frame in which to do so; or a feeling such as peace of mind, contentment, positiveness or any other mental state that you wish to achieve. Anything is possible!

Here is what you do.

## FORMULATING YOUR 'I' STATEMENTS

*Exercise:*
*Take a sheet of paper and define precisely what it is that you want to achieve. Keep the description as short and as simple as possible. The formula that you should use is similar to all the other 'I' statements that you have been repeating in the past six weeks. The golden rules are:*

- Keep it simple and accurate.
- Your statement should contain no negative words such as 'try' or 'hope', but only positive words that tell your subconscious that there is no possibility that you cannot achieve what it is that you want.
- Your statement should not contain more than two different ambitions, unless they are each associated directly with one another.

*When you have formulated that statement, repeat this over and over for ten minutes at the end of your five-minute pre-programming exercise and then spend another five minutes visualising how everything will be when you have achieved that aim. Make certain that you visualise and experience this with all of your senses and, at the appropriate moment, touch the tip of your little finger and thumb together and squeeze the picture gently into your subconscious mind.*

## KEEP A SCRAPBOOK

If it is material things that you seek in the future and you are determined to acquire them, your 'I' statement should be phrased in such a way that you already own this possession, even though you may only achieve ownership in the future.

For example, if it was a new house that you wished to move to, your statement should include the words 'I already own this home'.

Your visualisation exercise should then be carried out so that you describe in detail every aspect of this possession. You should see the outside of the house and the precise shape and structure of the building. You should visualise the colour of the walls and the paintwork, see the design and colour of the curtains hanging in the windows, the colour of the window frames and any other detail that you can imagine and that appeals to you.

You should see the gardens as they are planted and, if you find it necessary, you should even extend the time of your visualisation exercise and go into the house. See all the rooms fitted out and decorated exactly as you want them to be. You should feel the experiences that you are going to have in the future and hear the sounds that you associate with living there.

Suppose it was a new car that you wanted. If that is the case, you need to know the make, the model, the precise colour of the paintwork and the upholstery. You need to be able to visualise every detail inside and out and picture yourself clearly at the wheel. You also need to experience the feelings that you associate with owning and driving the car and hear the sounds that you will hear when you have it.

If it is a new partner that you seek in your life, I can assure you that if you use these same techniques, you will find that partner.

By carrying out your visualisation exercises in such detail you will programme your subconscious mind to make you take the physical steps that are necessary, without fear, in order to fulfil all your dreams and ambitions.

In addition to your visualisation exercises, you should keep a scrapbook and fill it with pictures of everything that you want for you and your family. Find pictures that fit your dream precisely and keep them in your book. This is one of the first steps towards making them a reality. The other steps will follow automatically. On the front of your scrapbook, write in large letters, 'These I Already Own'.

There is no more that I can do for you other than wish you a long, happy and fulfilling life. I hope that you enjoy it as much as I have enjoyed putting this programme together for you. I leave you with one final expression of my own:

*Success and achievement are your born rights,*
*not prizes for suffering.*

# Appendix

Eating Disorders and Other Behavioural Problems

Spot-reducing and Body-toning Exercises

A Seven-Day Menu Plan

Nutritional Support for Physical and Emotional
Problems

Best Food Sources of Nutrients

Recommended Reading on Nutrition and
Nutritional Therapy

How To Find a Qualified Nutritional Therapist

## EATING DISORDERS AND OTHER
## BEHAVIOURAL PROBLEMS

If there is one thing that I really feel uncomfortable with,
it is giving a medical or psychiatric problem a specific
name. For some reason, it always seems to make the
problem seem an awful lot worse.

So you have an eating disorder; that is why you turned
to this section of the programme. Whatever it is, I may
have the solution for you.

### Exercise:
*The following PDP exercise has helped many people in a similar situation to yourself and is very helpful in changing unhealthy and unwanted behavioural patterns. Do try this for a few days and see if it helps you. If you happen to be one of the few people who do not respond to this mental exercise, do please seek help from a qualified professional. There are a lot of people who can help you. If you find this necessary, do continue with this programme as well. It will act as a valuable support in dealing with your problem.*

*Find yourself a quiet, safe place where you will not be disturbed for fifteen minutes or so. Sit yourself in a comfortable chair and take several long, deep breaths and relax yourself.*

### Stage One
*Now I want you to identify clearly the behaviour that you want to change. Close your eyes and try to create a picture of you doing whatever it is that you want to stop doing. You may feel more able to create this picture as if it were a snapshot or you may wish to create it as if it were a film.*

*In either case, create it as brightly and vividly in your mind as you can. If it will have more impact on you as a black-and-white picture or film, see it in black and white. If the picture is more realistic in colour and you can picture it in colour, then make it coloured. Make this picture as vivid in your mind as it is possible to do.*

**Stage Two**
Now you need to create an entirely different picture in your mind. This picture is a picture of yourself as you would be if you no longer had this behavioural problem or eating disorder. Once again the picture can be a still or a film and can be in black and white or in colour. Put as much effort as you can into creating a scene or scenes which will represent exactly how you will be. Make certain that it includes all the very best and most appealing features you will have when you have made the change. Make this picture as clear as possible.

**Stage Three**
This is where you switch one picture for another in your conscious and subconscious mind and this is how you do it.

First of all, make a large, vivid picture of the behaviour that you want to change as you did in Stage One. Next, in the bottom right-hand corner of this picture, make a small, dark version of the picture of how you want to be as you did in Stage Two.

Now you do the switch. Take the small picture and, in a fraction of a second, blow it up in size. Make it bright and vivid and see it in your mind bursting through your first picture and exploding on to the screen in your mind. As you do this and as the second picture bursts through the screen, say out loud in a powerful voice 'WOW' and hold that new picture for at least five seconds.

Now open your eyes and close them again straight away

*and repeat Stage Three again for a total of ten times. Open your eyes for a second between each switch and do these switches as quickly as you possibly can. Do not forget that every time the new picture bursts through the old picture, you say 'WOW' with power.*

Every time you feel that your eating disorder is rearing its ugly head again, repeat these ten switch exercises. You could find that the problem may have vanished after only one session or it may take several in order for the cure to be permanent. Give this a week before deciding that you need help from another source unless the problem is causing you to feel abnormally unwell or has become life-threatening.

**Important Note**
You can use these switch exercises to change all sorts of behavioural problems other than eating disorders. I have used them successfully with patients to change a variety of bad habits and other problems, including nail-biting, smoking, phobias, frustrations, depression and numerous other negative mental attitudes.

## SPOT-REDUCING AND BODY-TONING EXERCISES

Many of you will be familiar with exercise routines and will have taken part in organised programmes at your local gymnasium or work-out and keep-fit studios. There are also several excellent books and videos on the market that will serve as refreshers for the experienced person and guides to those who have not exercised regularly before.

For those of you who are familiar with exercise programmes and particularly those aimed at reducing, toning and strengthening particular areas of the body, the following exercise routines will serve as an adequate reminder of what you need to do to sort out the major problem areas that need that extra help.

For those of you who are unfamiliar with exercise programmes, do not attempt to do these exercises without proper tuition and guidance. Incorrect or inadequate warm-up routines and incorrect posture whilst carrying out these exercises can do more harm than good.

### Spot-reducing for the Stomach and the Waist

#### 1 Curl-ups

Lie on your back on the floor with your knees bent at approximately right angles and with the soles of your feet flat on the floor. Put your hands behind your head and interlock your fingers.

Now, keeping your elbows pointed sideways, curl your upper body towards your knees until you are in an almost upright position. Breathe out as you do this. Hold for three seconds and return to a lying position. Repeat this exercise ten times.

Do this exercise twice a day.

### 2 Leg Lifts

Lie on your back on the floor, knees bent at approximately right angles, and rest your hands on your stomach.

Keeping your knees bent, raise both legs off the floor and bring them towards your chest. Then return them to the floor. If you find this exercise difficult, it is just as effective if you bring one leg at a time up towards the chest and do this alternately with each leg. Repeat this exercise ten times or ten times for each leg.

Do this series twice a day.

## Spot-reducing for the Bottom

### 1 Sit-stand Routine

Sit almost on the edge of an upright chair which has no arms. Your lower legs should be at right angles to your thighs and your feet should be firmly on the floor and about nine inches apart.

Now, without using your arms, just stand up from the chair into an upright position. Sit back down and repeat this twenty times.

Do this exercise twice a day.

## 2 Bottom Lifts

Kneel with your knees on the floor and your body in an upright position and look straight ahead. Keep your hands behind your back.

Now bend forward from the hips, keeping your upper legs as straight as possible, until your head touches the floor.

Using your bottom muscles, pull yourself up to the original starting position and repeat this fifteen times.

Do this series twice a day.

### Spot-reducing for the Hips and Thighs

#### 1 The Leg Raise

Lie on the floor on your left side and have your upper body supported on your left forearm and your right hand placed in front of you. Your hips should be squared facing forward. Next, bend your right leg and place the sole of your foot on the top of your left knee.

Now raise your left leg off the floor whilst using your right foot to exert pressure against the movement. Repeat the same exercise with the right and left leg positions reversed. Do this ten times with each leg.

Repeat the series twice a day.

## 2 *The Thigh Squeeze*

Lie flat on your back, your knees bent at approximately ninety degrees and your feet two to three inches apart. Next, slide your thighs open as far as is possible so that you arrive in a position with the soles of your feet touching each other.

Now, keeping your arms loose on the floor, bring up your thighs in a strong movement and squeeze them together, at the same time lifting your neck and upper back off the floor. Repeat this exercise fifteen times.

Do this exercise twice a day.

## Firming and Toning Bust and Chest Muscles

Sit in an upright chair with your neck and back very straight.

Hold your arms in front of you and grip the underside area of your lower arm, just above the wrist, with your opposite hand.

Gently push the skin up your arms with your hands and hold for two seconds, then relax. You will feel your chest muscles jump if you are doing this correctly.

Repeat this exercise ten to fifteen times every day.

## A SEVEN-DAY MENU PLAN

As I have mentioned earlier, there is no room in your programme either now, or at any time in the future, for any type of fad diets, replacement meals or anything that does not represent sensible and nutritious eating patterns.

Whilst there is no substitute for freshly prepared, wholesome food, I appreciate that this is not always possible, and there are some excellent, pre-packaged meals available in supermarkets which are designed for weight-conscious people.

For those readers who are not sure what constitutes sensible and nutritious eating patterns, and to save you interrupting this programme to rush out and buy a book that contains a variety of different menus and ideas for sensible meals, the following is a plan that you can follow for the next seven days or until you have acquired some other suitable reading material.

Please do bear in mind, however, that these suggestions take no account of foods that you have identified as creating additional cravings, and which should be avoided if mentioned here.

If you believe that you are carbohydrate intolerant, select those meals that contain the least amount of this food group or select those carbohydrate items which you believe have the least adverse effect upon you.

There are no quantities listed for the foods in any of these meals. Your subconscious mind knows how much you should be eating. Take notice of it when preparing your portions.

## Breakfast Suggestions
Choose from any of the following:

Muesli with skimmed milk
Special K Cereal with skimmed milk
1 boiled or poached egg and a slice of bread or toast –
    preferably wholemeal
A bowl of chopped fresh fruit with low-fat yoghurt
A chopped banana with low-fat yoghurt
Porridge cooked with water and served with honey

## Lunch and Evening Meal Suggestions
Choose from any of the following:

Jacket potato filled with baked beans
Jacket potato filled with grated carrot, tomato and
    sweetcorn
Cottage cheese (low fat) and salad
Tuna in brine and salad
Prawns and salad
Sandwich (preferably wholemeal bread) with any lean
    meat and salad filling
Scrambled or soft/hard-boiled egg and salad
Breast of chicken and salad
Spaghetti with tomato or meat sauce and a salad
Fish baked with tomatoes and served with two types
    of vegetables
Grilled fish with tomatoes and two types of vegetables
Stir-fried chicken breast cooked with onions, red and
    green peppers and bean shoots and served with rice
    (preferably wholegrain/brown rice)

Grilled steak served with green vegetables
Grilled lamb cutlets served with green vegetables
Lamb or beef casserole and vegetables

*Notes:*
Vegetables should be prepared without fat.
Salads should be served without fat or with low-fat
   dressings.

**Desserts**
Fresh fruit
Frozen yoghurt
Low-fat ice cream
Stewed apples with honey
Stewed prunes with honey
Stewed rhubarb with honey

**Drinks**
Tea and coffee – as much as you want, but watch the milk
Low-calorie or no-calorie drinks – as much as you want

## NUTRITIONAL SUPPORT FOR PHYSICAL AND EMOTIONAL PROBLEMS

The following information will provide you with guidelines on how to support the problems listed with foods that contain the nutrients necessary to assist you, as well as with recommended food supplements. Foods that contain the highest and most appropriate levels of the nutrients listed are found at the end of this section.

Where no amount of the nutrient is listed, do not take supplements but emphasise the correct foods in your meal planning. These are listed on the following pages in this section. Doses of nutrients listed are the daily dose recommended.

**Whilst I wholeheartedly support and endorse the use of vitamin, mineral and other nutritional supplements, it is possible that some people may suffer an allergic reaction to various dietary supplements or the mediums in which they are prepared. If such reactions occur, then you must consult your doctor before continuing with such supplementation. Ideally, any programme of supplement support should be carried out under the guidance of a qualified person.**

Please also note that it is in every person's health interests to take a multi-vitamin and mineral supplement every day. If you do, you may find that the quantity of specific nutrient listed under the headings below is already included in the multi-vitamin and mineral supplement. If the quantity included is insufficient, you will need to take an additional supplement of that item.

## Alcohol

Whether you are carbohydrate intolerant or not, if you believe that alcohol is having or has had any detrimental effect on your body, you should abstain.

In addition, take the following supplements and select foods to eat that contain the nutrients listed.

| | |
|---|---|
| Vitamin A | 25,000 IU daily |
| Vitamin B Complex | Ask your pharmacist for a high-dose tablet |
| Vitamin C | 2000mg |
| Vitamin D | 1000 IU |
| Vitamin E | 1000 IU |
| Chromium | |
| Iron | |
| Manganese | 500mg |
| Magnesium | 500mg |
| Zinc | 150mg |
| Unsaturated fatty acids | |
| Glutamine | 1000mg 3 times daily |

## Brown Fat Cell Activation

The following nutrients will assist the activity of brown fat cells:

| | |
|---|---|
| Zinc | 20mg |
| Copper | 3mg |

## Constipation

There are numerous causes of constipation. Avoid chemical laxatives if possible; these only perpetuate the problem and can even make matters worse.

Emphasise more fibre in the diet from fruits, especially apples, papaya, pineapple, prunes and figs. Emphasise the use of vegetables and wholegrain cereals when making meals and drink plenty of water. Other foods that may help are garlic and yoghurt.

## Diarrhoea

Because food passes through the system far too quickly with this condition, the body does not have time to absorb many of the essential nutrients contained in the food which can have an effect on all other systems in the body. In addition, a great deal of essential water is lost from the body.

Recommended supplements are:

| | |
|---|---|
| Vitamin A | 25,000 IU |
| Vitamin B Complex | Ask your pharmacist for a high-dose tablet |
| Vitamin C | 2000mg |
| Calcium | 2000mg |
| Iron | |
| Magnesium | 500mg |
| Potassium | |
| Sodium | |
| Acidophilus | |

## Low Energy and Fatigue

If you have low energy levels and fatigue, you must exercise in moderation and balance this with periods of adequate rest as well as eating for full nutritional support.

Recommended supplements are:

| | |
|---|---|
| Vitamin A | 25,000 IU |
| Vitamin B Complex | Ask your pharmacist for a high-dose tablet |
| Folic Acid | |
| Vitamin C | 2000mg |
| Vitamin D | |
| Iron | |
| Magnesium | 50mg |
| Manganese | |
| Potassium | |

## Metabolic Test

If your results were on the low side, follow the programme for activating brown fat cells.

**Stress**
A certain amount of stress is useful as a motivating factor, but excess stress is detrimental to your entire body. Nutrients that support this condition are:

| | |
|---|---|
| Vitamin A | 25,000 IU |
| Vitamin B Complex | Ask your pharmacist for a high-dose tablet |
| Vitamin C | 2000mg |
| Vitamin D | |
| Vitamin E | |
| Calcium | 500mg |
| Chromium | |
| Copper | |
| Iodine | |
| Iron | |
| Magnesium | 100mg |
| Manganese | |
| Potassium | |
| Selenium | |
| Zinc | |

# BEST FOOD SOURCES OF NUTRIENTS

## Vitamin A
Liver
Eggs
Yellow fruits and vegetables
Dark green fruits and vegetables
Fish-liver oil

## Vitamin B
Brewer's yeast
Whole grains
Brown rice
Meat, fish and poultry
Legumes
Eggs
Dark green leafy vegetables
Citrus fruits
Yoghurt

## Vitamin C
Citrus fruits
Kiwi fruit
Sprouted alfalfa seeds
Strawberries
Broccoli
Tomatoes
Green peppers

**Vitamin D**
Fish and fish-liver oils
Egg yolks
Organ meats (liver or kidney)

**Vitamin E**
Eggs
Wheatgerm
Organ meats
Leafy vegetables

**Folic Acid**
Dark green leafy vegetables
Organ meats
Root vegetables
Whole grains
Oysters
Milk

**Calcium**
Milk and milk products
Green leafy vegetables
Shellfish

**Chromium**
Honey
Grapes
Raisins
Wholegrain cereals

**Copper**
Organ meats
Seafood
Nuts
Raisins
Legumes

**Iron**
Organ meats
Eggs
Fish
Poultry
Green leafy vegetables
Dried fruit

**Magnesium**
Seafood
Whole grains
Dark green vegetables

**Manganese**
Whole grains
Green leafy vegetables
Legumes
Pineapple
Egg yolk

**Potassium**
Lean meat
Vegetables
Whole grains
Dried fruit
Legumes

**Selenium**
Tuna
Herring
Whole grains
Wheatgerm and wheat bran

**Sodium**
Seafood
Table salt
Celery
Milk products

**Zinc**
Organ meats
Seafood
Mushrooms
Soybeans
Eggs
Wheatgerm

**Acidophilus**
Natural live yoghurt

**Glutamine and Tyrosine**
Cereals and grains
Eggs
Fruits
Seafood
Poultry
Vegetables
Nuts and seeds

# RECOMMENDED READING ON NUTRITION AND NUTRITIONAL THERAPY

*Nutrition Almanac* by John D. Kirschmann
Published by McGraw-Hill

*Nutritional Medicine* by Davis and Stewart
Published by Pan

*Diet and Nutrition* by Ballentine
Published by Himmalayan

*Diet for a New World* by John Robbins
Published by Avon

You may also wish to study this subject by correspondence. An excellent course is run by The International College of Natural Health Sciences, 2 Bath Place, Rivington Street, London EC2A 3JJ, Tel: 0171-454 9988.

## HOW TO FIND A QUALIFIED NUTRITIONAL THERAPIST

*Contact:*
The British Naturopathic Association
Frazer House, 6 Netherhall Gardens, London NW3 5RR

Incorporated Society of Registered Naturopaths
328 Harrowgate Road, Leeds LS17 6PE

# SUPER JUICE FOR SLIMMERS

### Over 150 juicing recipes to help you lose weight and stay healthy

## BEVERLEY PIPER

## SUPER JUICE FOR SLIMMERS

shows you how to use invigorating live juice as part of your weight-watching programme.

Fruit and vegetable juices are a real boon to slimmers: not only are they quick and easy to make, but they are delicious and low in calories too! They are also bursting with essential vitamins and minerals, and will help to boost energy levels and promote sensible slimming.

All the recipes are calorie counted and you can choose from a wide range of nutritious drink and tasty meal ideas. Try, for example, a refreshing cocktail of carrot, pineapple and cucumber juice or an appetising dish of chicken in plum and orange sauce.

Complete with 10 specially designed seven-day diet plans, SUPER JUICE FOR SLIMMERS brings you an exciting new way to lose weight and stay healthy.

'Juicing is deeply tempting to anyone who struggles with a weight problem' *Daily Mail*

**NON-FICTION/HEALTH/DIET   0 7472 4573 8**

# A selection of non-fiction from Headline

| | | |
|---|---|---|
| THE DRACULA SYNDROME | Richard Monaco & William Burt | £5.99 ☐ |
| DEADLY JEALOUSY | Martin Fido | £5.99 ☐ |
| WHITE COLLAR KILLERS | Frank Jones | £4.99 ☐ |
| THE MURDER YEARBOOK 1994 | Brian Lane | £5.99 ☐ |
| THE PLAYFAIR CRICKET ANNUAL | Bill Frindall | £3.99 ☐ |
| ROD STEWART | Stafford Hildred & Tim Ewbank | £5.99 ☐ |
| THE JACK THE RIPPER A–Z | Paul Begg, Martin Fido & Keith Skinner | £7.99 ☐ |
| THE DAILY EXPRESS HOW TO WIN ON THE HORSES | Danny Hall | £4.99 ☐ |
| COUPLE SEXUAL AWARENESS | Barry & Emily McCarthy | £5.99 ☐ |
| GRAPEVINE: THE COMPLETE WINEBUYERS HANDBOOK | Anthony Rose & Tim Atkins | £5.99 ☐ |
| ROBERT LOUIS STEVENSON: DREAMS OF EXILE | Ian Bell | £7.99 ☐ |

*All Headline books are available at your local bookshop or newsagent, or can be ordered direct from the publisher. Just tick the titles you want and fill in the form below. Prices and availability subject to change without notice.*

Headline Book Publishing, Cash Sales Department, Bookpoint, 39 Milton Park, Abingdon, OXON, OX14 4TD, UK. If you have a credit card you may order by telephone – 0235 400400.

Please enclose a cheque or postal order made payable to Bookpoint Ltd to the value of the cover price and allow the following for postage and packing:
UK & BFPO: £1.00 for the first book, 50p for the second book and 30p for each additional book ordered up to a maximum charge of £3.00.
OVERSEAS & EIRE: £2.00 for the first book, £1.00 for the second book and 50p for each additional book.

Name .........................................................................................................

Address ......................................................................................................

....................................................................................................................

....................................................................................................................

If you would prefer to pay by credit card, please complete:
Please debit my Visa/Access/Diner's Card/American Express (delete as applicable) card no:

| | | | | | | | | | | | | | | | |
|---|---|---|---|---|---|---|---|---|---|---|---|---|---|---|---|
| | | | | | | | | | | | | | | | |

Signature ............................................................ Expiry Date .........